Praise for *Blast from the Past*

"This book tells fascinating stories about connections into other lifetimes that have an influence on this one. The messages behind Shelley's work are both clear and powerful. Not only do we live many times and there is nothing to fear from death, but we can learn so much from these journeys into other lives. This book will help you start that journey."

—Peter Smith, author of *Quantum Consciousness*

"This book is a gem and I believe contributes not only to the past life regression field of study, but also offers an effective alternative and efficacious supplement to the internal healing process. All events and relationships, whether past or future or present, coexist, awaiting our re-cognition and our love in the form of acceptance and letting go. Shelley's book verifies this need within every human being—whether they are aware of this need or not—and her book comes up with the goods to guide this process."

—Neale Lundgren, PhD, author of
Meditations for the Soul

"What a wonderful collection of insightful stories and guided journeys Dr. Shelley A. Kaehr offers us in *Blast from the Past*! Each is an opportunity to learn how experiences and relationships in this lifetime relate to our own Soul's Purposes."

—Dr. Linda Howe, Akashic Records expert,
teacher and author of *Inspired Manifesting*

"*Blast from the Past* could be retitled 'Everything You Wanted to Know about Reincarnation but Were Afraid to Ask.' It is one of the most comprehensive and fascinating books on reincarnation that I have ever read and it's full of useful ideas to understand and to explore the effects of past-life experiences."

—Kenneth J Doka, PhD, author of *When We Die*

"We've all had [spontaneous recalls]. We touch an object or gemstone, come across a place or a person, and we're suddenly engaged in a 'yesterday' that holds either a pleasant or unpleasant remembering. *Blast from the Past* is the first book I've ever read that helps you recognize these unprompted experiences and use them to transform and heal. An amazing resource of discussions, case studies, and exercises designed to help you courageously look behind so you can confidently step forward."

—Cyndi Dale, author of *Energy Healing*
for Trauma, Stress & Chronic Illness

"An amazing approach to showing us how we can discover where our current hurts, joys, blocks, talents, pains, tendencies, successes, and restrictions come from … Dr. Kaehr details how our past lives can reveal so much to us in our current and future lives. Figuring out our past existences without a regression session helps us to do the work in our private space and retrieve past knowledge that can help us flourish … Her book is packed with realizations and insights, and it's full of exercises and guidance we can use to contemplate the future by way of delving into the past … Well worth the read; this book is a gift."

—Kac Young PhD, ND, DCH, RScM,
author of *Crystal Power*

"Dr. Shelley Kaehr demonstrates how bad vibes or weird feelings come from a place most of us never realized—our past lives. Dr. Kaehr shows readers how to alleviate these situations with guided imagery and helpful exercises. Highly recommended to all struggling to make sense of our weird world."

—George Noory, host of Coast to Coast AM

"From top to bottom, Shelley Kaehr's latest book *Blast from the Past* hits on all cylinders…The depth, clarity, and quality of the information, examples, testimonials, and clearly outlined exercises make this book an amazing tool to release yourself from generational and lifetime energies that are impacting your current reality…Definitely a great book to have in your toolbox!"

—R. James Case, author of *Fear Is a Choice*
and host of *The Adventures in Truth* podcast

BLAST
from the
PAST

About the Author

For two decades, **Shelley A. Kaehr, PhD** (Dallas, TX), has worked with thousands of people around the world, helping them achieve greater peace and happiness in their lives. A world-renowned past life regressionist, Dr. Shelley's method of combining energy work with hypnosis has been endorsed by numerous leaders in the field of consciousness, including near-death experience pioneers Dr. Raymond Moody and Dr. Brian Weiss. Dr. Shelley has been prominently featured in the media, including *Coast to Coast AM* and William Shatner's *Weird or What*. She received her PhD in Parapsychic Science from the American Institute of Holistic Theology in 2001.

Connect with Dr. Shelley A. Kaehr:
Website: https://pastlifelady.com
Facebook Fan Page: Past Life Lady
Instagram: shelleykaehr
YouTube: Past Life Lady
Twitter: @ShelleyKaehr

SHELLEY A. KAEHR, PhD

BLAST

from the

PAST

Healing Spontaneous
Past Life Memories

Llewellyn Publications
Woodbury, Minnesota

FIRST EDITION
First Printing, 2021

Book design by Sammy Peterson
Cover design by Shira Atakpu

Llewellyn Publications is a registered trademark of Llewellyn Worldwide Ltd.

Library of Congress Cataloging-in-Publication Data
Names: Kaehr, Shelley, author.
Title: Blast from the past : healing spontaneous past life memories /
    Shelley A. Kaehr, PhD.
Description: First edition. | Woodbury, Minnesota : Llewellyn Publications,
    [2021] | Includes bibliographical references.
Identifiers: LCCN 2021039611 | ISBN 9780738768502 (paperback) | ISBN
    9780738768700 (ebook)
Subjects: LCSH: Reincarnation. | Memory. | Déjà vu.
Classification: LCC BL515 .K328 2021 | DDC 133.901/35—dc23
LC record available at https://lccn.loc.gov/2021039611

Llewellyn Worldwide Ltd. does not participate in, endorse, or have any authority or responsibility concerning private business transactions between our authors and the public.

All mail addressed to the author is forwarded but the publisher cannot, unless specifically instructed by the author, give out an address or phone number.

Any internet references contained in this work are current at publication time, but the publisher cannot guarantee that a specific location will continue to be maintained. Please refer to the publisher's website for links to authors' websites and other sources.

Llewellyn Publications
A Division of Llewellyn Worldwide Ltd.
2143 Wooddale Drive
Woodbury, MN 55125-2989
www.llewellyn.com

Printed in the United States of America

Other Books by Shelley A. Kaehr, PhD

Beyond Reality: Evidence of Parallel Universes

Familiar Places: Reflections on Past Lives Around the World

Heal Your Ancestors to Heal Your Life:
The Transformative Power of Genealogical Regression

Lifestream: Journey into Past & Future Lives

Meet Your Karma: The Healing Power of Past Life Memories

Past Lives with Gems & Stones

Past Lives with Pets: Discover Your Timeless
Connection to Your Beloved Companions

Reincarnation Recollections: Geographically Induced Past Life Memories

Supretrovie: Externally Induced Past Life Memories

CONTENTS

EXERCISES

Chapter Six

DISCLAIMER

This book is not intended as a substitute for consultation with a licensed medical or mental health professional. The reader should regularly consult a physician or mental health professional in matters relating to their health and particularly with respect to any symptoms that may require diagnosis or medical attention. This book provides content related to educational, medical, and psychological topics. As such, use of this book implies your acceptance of this disclaimer.

Names and identifying details have been changed to protect the privacy of individuals.

ACKNOWLEDGMENTS

Gratitude and extreme kudos to the incomparable Angela Wix, who encouraged me to write this book. Thank you! I also owe an extreme debt of gratitude to Bill Krause, Terry Lohmann, Kat Sanborn, and Anna Levine, who helped me expand my audience by providing online forums for my content during the global lockdown. Thank you all for being amazing publishing partners! To Lauryn Heineman, Andy Belmas, Shannon McKuhen, Sami Sherratt, Jake-Ryan Kent, Alisha Bjorklund, Lynne Menturweck, Patti Frazee, Kevin Brown, Donna Burch-Brown, Annie Burdick, Leah Madsen, Sammy Peterson, and the rest of the Llewellyn team, I simply cannot thank you enough for your help and support on this and all my Llewellyn titles. To my family and friends, thanks for sticking by me all these years through the ups and downs of life. Special thanks to Jim Merideth, Pat Moon, and Paula Wagner. Above all, I thank my students and clients, who continue to be completely awe-inspiring.

FOREWORD

I FOUND A KINDRED spirit in Shelley Kaehr when I was introduced to her through our publisher to be a guest on her show. I began to read her books and discovered we shared many common beliefs about hypnosis, regression, and energy and the connection between them, though we had never met prior to my interview with her. In her latest book, Shelley insightfully shares client case histories as well as her own regarding Supretrovie, a term she's coined to describe spontaneous past life memories arising from objects, people, and places. This is a topic that's often overlooked or not written about.

What I especially appreciate is the way Shelley breaks down the subtle differences between the various trance-inducing memory recall states to help the reader identify each state and recognize their own experiences with Supretrovie. She also gives valuable insights on how to heal from those experiences.

The exercises provided in part 2 are a wonderful way for the reader to open up and discover new or remember old instances of Supretrovie in their own lives. Some instances of Supretrovie may be merely reminders of the past, while others may need resolution with the help of a qualified regressionist.

According to Shelley, when a Supretrovie comes to the surface, it's time for something to be resolved. I've found this to be true in my own private practice. My clients are frequently prompted to seek me out after experiencing remarkable spontaneous past life memories that emerge during trips, around objects, or upon first meeting people. We explore through regression to uncover more details behind the Supretrovie and, most importantly, to release unpleasant experiences to neutralize their effects on the client moving forward. We also look at the benefits of the experience and how it can help the client.

I've had many of my own experiences with Supretrovie, too! I recall one experience when I was traveling through the London Heathrow Airport and suddenly felt physically ill. My traveling companions were all fine, but I couldn't wait for my several-hour layover to be over. When it was finally over and we were well on our way to Spain, I immediately felt better. It was years later when I was studying hypnosis, specifically regression therapy, that I explored that memory further to discover I had had a past life as an artist near there.

It was in 1600 London. My parents, who were very poor, made the tough decision to leave me in apprenticeship to a local artist, thinking they were giving me an opportunity and helping the family with one less mouth to feed. I was a young boy of about ten years old, and they had been told that the artist would teach me how to paint like him. I looked forward to learning from a respected artist.

Once my father dropped me off with him and a tiny sum of money exchanged in trade for me, I soon realized things weren't as we had been led to believe. The place we lived in was dimly lit with one stone left out of the exterior wall to let light in. Candles were expensive, so he painted in the makeshift window while daylight lasted. I was made to stand in the corner out of his way—having a pitcher of water, bread, and cheese ready when he requested them—and clean up after him when he was finished painting for the day. He mocked and scolded me constantly. I ate the crumbs he left behind. My clothes were tattered and dirty. I slept on the cold, hard stone floor with only a thin piece of fabric to cover me at night. There were no art lessons, though sometimes I played with his left-over paints before cleaning them up. I was merely a servant and was very unhappy there.

I did learn to paint—not because of him, but because of me. I learned by watching him all those years. Endless hours of watching him and waiting on him taught me patience and to observe. When he died, I had no life skills. I tried to make it on my own as an artist and lasted a short time, eventually dying of starvation, penniless, lying in the streets.

What's interesting is that I recognized this person in my current life as an artist, too—one of my early acting teachers. I began to understand better why I wanted to look up to him but never completely trusted him (and with good reason). In some ways, I was afraid of him, thinking that he held the keys to my success in his hands. He presented himself as someone who had connections in the industry, as if he had the power to make me or break me. He seemingly enjoyed chiding me in class whenever he was in a mood. It also explained a nagging feeling I had of ending in peril if I pursued a career in the arts ... which I eventually got past, clearing up that Supretrovie for good!

This time around, I learned from him as an actor and enjoyed pushing boundaries through scene work, but most importantly, he helped me by teaching me to stand up for myself against him. When it all came down, the man I thought I could learn from taught me the most by my finding the courage to walk away. I stood up for myself and used that to move on, carving my own way in the field and making my own contacts along the way.

Clients seek out sessions to further explore feelings or even visions that have happened when visiting a particular place sparks a sense of deep familiarity and emotional response that often linger long after the event. That's when the regression session can be helpful to bring more information to the client's conscious awareness, resolve the issue, and bring understanding.

One client's experience of Supretrovie happened in layers, beginning during a group past life regression I was facilitating for a documentary a couple of years ago. In the group experience, she went to a past life in what she believed to be the Middle East: a sandy village where she was a gay man who was persecuted for wanting to be with his lover. He died for the lover and because of their love.

She told me after the group regression that although she loved to venture on her own and travel to foreign lands, the past life details didn't "resonate." She was more struck by how she felt heat behind her back and a fire the entire time of that regression. She asked me if there had ever been a fire here at the Braithe Center. I replied, "Yes, there used to be a fireplace along the wall you were sitting against that caught fire several years before I moved in. When they rebuilt, the entire fireplace was taken out." She just looked at me in astonishment.

Fast-forward to 2020, when COVID hit. Not long before this, my client was introduced to a man who loves to travel as much as she does. He was already out of the country. They texted a few times and made plans to meet up in Ukraine, but by then European countries were shutting down due to COVID. Within a few hours of departure, they decided to meet up on the West Coast of Africa instead.

His voice messages were beginning to stir feelings of "love" for this man she barely knew, as if "he was the one," she later wrote me. Just as strong were feelings of having been to the West Coast before when she landed and stepped out into the sand and sun. It was all too familiar.

She explored a bit while she waited in the village for him to arrive. She heard her name being called out, immediately recognizing the voice from the messages. She shared with me that "as soon as I hugged him, my soul knew, knew, *knew* that some healing was about to happen."

She quickly realized that although they had a connection, it wasn't the same for him as it was for her. It didn't matter, though. They got on well and ended up living together in this African village due to COVID for a couple of months. My client was elated at being given the chance to "play 'house,' be in a 'relationship,' and say her peace with the soul of this man." When she eventually told him about their past life together, he was interested, but he seemed rather indifferent about it. For her, this was a wonderful way to work out what her soul had longed for with his soul hundreds of years ago. She also spent a great deal of time getting reacquainted with her past in the village. "But as you know … the soul knows," she said.

These stories are fascinating, but I'm not so surprised. The twists and turns that take place in our lives to reconnect with people from our past, regardless of geographical location, are amazing. And yes, the soul does know!

Bryn Blankinship, CMHt, CI
The Regression Specialist©
Author of *The Limitless Soul: Hypno-Regression*
Case Studies into Past, Present & Future Lives

INTRODUCTION

EVER SINCE CHILDHOOD WHEN I first became aware of the concept of reincarnation, I believed in it as my personal truth. In adulthood, after receiving a powerful past life regression that helped me fully resolve years of grief, I realized this would become my life's calling—to help others heal from the effects of their past.

I've been working in the field now for over twenty years. I used to believe that people needed to have a regression to successfully locate the time periods where certain unwanted influences originated. Not anymore. A few years ago, my understanding shifted after a series of weird events caused me to rethink my philosophies and come to terms with the reality that people do not need to undergo hypnosis to remember, but rather to *heal* from the onslaught of sensations that often come up from out of nowhere without warning.

As a lifelong wanderer, the idea of spontaneous past life recall from travel first occurred to me back in 2006. After teaching throughout the US that year and traveling to Russia, I made notes in my journal about my idea that the soul must be attempting to reconnect with former experiences through travel. Like most people, I am often motivated through pain and unpleasant experiences, which is why it took several more years and a jolting experience to make me pursue that line of reasoning more seriously.

In 2013, I purchased a travel agency and took groups on tours to various places around the world. On a cruise to Key West, although the beauty of the gorgeous little town struck me, I left feeling that either allergens in the air made me ill or that the place itself must be cursed. Once our ship floated far enough away from land, I suddenly felt so much better. I convinced myself that the problem must be the latter. As a lifelong optimist, I didn't want to conclude that any place was cursed. I believe we create reality with our thoughts. Still, I couldn't help but think that had to be the case. Key West had bad vibes, period, so I vowed never to return. I've explored the strength of vows in other writings, and often when we are so adamant about our positions in life, trouble ensues, and these places often give clues to hidden issues that need to be resolved within the soul. At the time, I hadn't yet recognized that fact. Rather than thinking I should look within, I could only consider that the place itself had a problem.

A week or so after returning from the trip, out of the blue, friends invited me to return to Key West. At first, I said no. There would be absolutely no way I would go back to a place that made me feel so miserable. Once I finished objecting, I started to become curious and realized the universe must have some reason for presenting the opportunity to me so soon, and I thought that perhaps it would be a good idea to take a closer look at why Key West made me so unhappy.

I asked one of my past life regression students to help me find answers. Sure enough, I went back into my former lifetime in the 1600s when I worked as a deckhand on a ship. I managed to anger the captain and crew so badly, they tossed me overboard after a walk down the plank. I struggled to shore and perished right in the spot where I had experienced a horrible reaction during my recent trip.

After going through my regression, I had a deep curiosity to see whether or not the regression would really work to resolve my issues so I could at least get through the day without becoming ill.

I returned to Key West, and although I had an initial feeling of being ill, I used the tools you're going to read about in this book to help me move through the challenge and actually come very close to the exact place where I believe I perished in that past life. Once I did some healing on the past, I went around the gorgeous city for the remainder of my time there and had a wonderful adventure. Thanks to all of this, I now have a special place in my heart for the quirky little town of Key West.

Through this experience, I began recalling other times when I had either horrible experiences or especially pleasant times while traveling. I realized that both are indicative of past life memories bleeding through to the current lifetime.

The profound healing I received personally led me to question other people about whether or not they had ever experienced such things, and to my surprise, I realized these kinds of situations are incredibly common. This book is the product of my belief that this phenomenon, which I call *Supretrovie*, happens to people all the time, whether they're aware of it or not. I became convinced that much of our daily experience is colored by things that happened to us long ago, and by and large, most people are not at all aware of what's happening. You have a bad experience, and you simply close the door on it, like I almost did, and move on with your life. That makes sense, but what if you could have a more neutral and peaceful experience by bringing conscious awareness to these issues? By providing case histories and suggestions for healing, I truly believe this book will help you bring greater joy, peace, and stability to your life journey.

Supretrovie Overview

For years I have endorsed the idea that past life regression helps people uncover memories that can be healed to experience greater happiness in life. *What if you could discover your past lives without a regression?*

After I became consciously aware of how the past affects the present, I've since encountered hundreds of people who have spontaneously recalled past life memories while traveling or being in the presence of certain objects, artifacts, or people. Instead of using regression for discovery, the modality is used for transformative healing. After discovering the widespread prevalence of this phenomenon, I coined the term *Supretrovie*. The word combines *retro*, a word that indicates moving backward into the past, with the French *vie*, meaning life, and the Latin/French/English prefix *super*, which means beyond, above, or fantastical, because these memories originate from a supernatural source, beyond the realm of our five rational senses.

What you will likely discover is that the answer to the question above is a resounding yes. Not only can you discover your past lives without a regression, you've probably already been doing so outside of your conscious awareness. It's highly likely that as you review this information and the case histories in part 2, you will recall events from your life that reflect unexpected feelings or thoughts you've had, and you'll realize that the events are most likely related to a long-forgotten memory of one of your past lives. Sounds exciting, right?

Comparing Supretrovie to Other Phenomenon

Before we fully dive into the material in *Blast from the Past*, I must explain how Supretrovie differs from other paranormal phenomenon. I've devoted several years to this research to raise awareness about a largely subconscious and often unpleasant reaction we've all had to places and things so that we might gain greater understanding of what's really happening and create greater peace and happiness in our lives. To that point, I feel it's important to share more details about my research and explain why the phenomenon of Supretrovie differs from other common occurrences in paranormal research.

In prior books, I defined Supretrovie based on only two kinds of occurrences, but after receiving extensive feedback from so many who reported these paranormal happenings, I've expanded my definition of Supretrovie to include one of four criteria:

1. Geographically induced from travel. The subject is in a new location and suddenly recalls a previous incarnation. Modern sur-

roundings often fade away, and the subject's interior mindscape is filled by a movie or vision of the way things appeared in the past.

2. Holding or being in close proximity to an artifact, antique, or object from a past life experience. This could be the exact item the subject owned before, or something reminiscent of the past.

3. Working with a gemstone or mineral that triggers a past life memory from the part of the world where the stone is from.

4. Meeting a person whom you knew in a past life and recalling previously unknown events where you interacted with that person.

Supretrovie often comes with certain symptoms that are quite common among experiencers, including the following:

- Dizziness
- Nausea
- Movies of unfamiliar settings running in the mind
- Modern features vanishing and being replaced in the mind by ancient settings
- Disorientation

My original writings did not go into the aspects of gems and stones or the undeniable connections we share with people we meet, but as of this writing and thanks to so many who responded to surveys I've sent out through the years, I believe these are important to include in this exploration. I conducted one of my surveys back in 2019 to ask my readers if they had ever experienced Supretrovie or similar paranormal phenomena. I've included the quiz here for you to take.

Past Life Memories Survey

1. Have you ever experienced déjà vu—the illusion of having previously experienced something actually being encountered for the first time? For example, you're having a chat with someone, and

you know you've had this same conversation earlier, although you have no idea when or why.

2. Have you ever experienced anamnesis—the recollection of ideas that the soul had known in a previous existence, especially by means of reasoning? For example, if you always knew you lived a prior life in England without having to go through a past life regression —a soul knowing.

3. Have you ever experienced Supretrovie—an externally induced past life memory triggered by travel? For example, let's say you travel to New York, and while you're walking around, you have a sudden visual image, thought, sound, or feeling of a time when you were there before that did not happen in your current lifetime.

4. Have you ever experienced Supretrovie triggered by an object? For example, you go to an antique store and pick up a necklace or other object and suddenly have a vision, thought, or feeling that you've owned the object before, or you recall a place and time long ago that are not part of your current life experience.

Here are the survey results I received from my 2019 survey:

100 percent experienced déjà vu.

83 percent had anamnesis or soul knowing about their prior lives.

67 percent had Supretrovie triggered by traveling.

84 percent experienced Supretrovie in the presence of an object.

Like me, you may be surprised to see how common such experiences are for many people. For years, I've consistently received feedback that showed a very high percentage of people have definitely had these experiences happen to them.

While Supretrovie is new, the idea of spontaneous recall and remembering our past without hypnosis is not. Let's take a closer look at each of the similar phenomena to further explore how these anomalies differ from Supretrovie.

Déjà Vu versus Supretrovie

My interpretation of déjà vu would be an event that happens in your current lifetime that has nothing to do with past lives. Usually a very mundane activity is recalled as though you did that same exact thing at an earlier time in your current life. A great example would be if you and I were out having dinner at a restaurant together, and during our conversation, we began having a feeling that the two of us had been in that exact same restaurant having that same exact conversation at some time in the past. We would feel as though we'd somehow glimpsed our future selves in the middle of this seemingly routine event.

That's one thing I've noticed about déjà vu. The scenes are never anything especially remarkable. They're simple and straightforward, and yet so profound in their nature to remind and trigger our subconscious minds to understand that this is something we've encountered before. Déjà vu can often feel like our spirit guides and helpers are shaking our shoulders and whispering in our ears, "Hey, this is important!" even when the actual content of the déjà vu isn't much to talk about. Our spirit guides test us to make sure we're paying attention, and déjà vu helps us practice listening.

Many of my students and clients have desperately wanted one thing—to enhance their intuition. They've felt frustrated they don't seem to be "getting" deeper connections to their spirit guides and unseen forces that would help them navigate the choppy waters of life. One point I always make is the fact that, in order to receive more information about such things, you have to acknowledge the little events: the seemingly unimportant occurrences that are small miracles but often go overlooked. A good analogy is seeking a job promotion. You want more money and greater responsibility, but first, you must learn to master the more mundane tasks. Déjà vu is our guides helping us experience the divine at a deeper level and is a wonderful test of spirit.

Because déjà vu typically involves replays of scenes from our current lifetimes that feel like memories and Supretrovie is triggered by external events, they're not at all the same. Rather than reliving modern times, people who have Supretrovie report modern surroundings fading away and memories of times in the deep past bubbling up from out of nowhere.

Plato's Anamnesis

Renowned philosopher Plato came up with the brilliant idea that the soul retains knowledge learned in prior lifetimes. The word *anamnesis* is derived from the Greek word meaning "recalling to mind."[1] Plato described this concept in his dialogues *Meno*, *Phaedo*, and *Phaedus*.

Dictionary.com defines *anamnesis* as "Platonism. Recollection of the Ideas, which the soul had known in a previous existence, especially by means of reasoning."[2]

In *Meno*, Plato argues the nature of knowledge with his character Socrates, who is based on his real-life teacher. He argues that if someone seeks knowledge, when they find it, they won't realize it, since they had no prior knowledge of the information. Socrates refutes this by telling Plato that a person's soul is filled with soul knowledge carried over from other incarnations:

"The soul, then, as being immortal, and having been born again many times, and having seen all things that exist, whether in this world or in the world below, has knowledge of them all; and it is no wonder that she should be able to call to remembrance all that she ever knew about virtue, and about everything; for as all nature is akin, and the soul has learned all things; there is no difficulty in her eliciting or as men say learning, out of

---

1. Encyclopaedia Britannica, "Anamnesis," *Encyclopaedia Britannica*, https://www.britannica.com/art/anamnesis.

2. Dictionary.com, "Anamnesis," *Dictionary.com*, https://www.dictionary.com/browse/anamnesis?s=t.

a single recollection—all the rest, if a man is strenuous and does not faint; for all enquiry and all learning is but recollection." [3]

Socrates explains the reason we do not recall what we did in prior lifetimes is because of the trauma of birth. He demonstrates this by asking a boy to recall geometry, and with proper questioning, the boy eventually finds the truth, which proves he knew the answer from another incarnation but forgot until Socrates helped him.

In *Phaedo*, Plato further explains how anamnesis can be achieved by contemplating issues with the soul, which is of a higher nature than the physical body:

"While in company with the body the soul cannot have pure knowledge, one of two things seems to follow—either knowledge is not to be attained at all, or, if at all, after death." [4]

In Plato's *Phaedrus*, he also describes the idea that the soul contains the totality of mind and knowledge:

"There abides the very being with which true knowledge is concerned; the colourless, formless, intangible essence, visible only to mind, the pilot of the soul." [5]

Anamnesis is quite real. I've run into plenty of people who know exactly who they were in the past. When somebody tells me they lived in England, for example, I always believe them. There's typically a confidence in their demeanor when relating information that comes from the soul level that cannot be denied.

Supretrovie differs from anamnesis because it is produced by an *external* source rather than simply sitting dormant in our minds. Something outside of the subject causes Supretrovie to happen beyond an inner soul knowing. The person had no awareness at all of the past life prior to the external event happening.

---

3. Benjamin Jowett, *MENO by Plato 380 BC* (New York: C. Scribner's Sons, 1871), 1.

4. Benjamin Jowett, *PHAEDO by Plato 360 BC* (New York: C. Scribner's Sons, 1871), 8.

5. Benjamin Jowett, *PHAEDRUS by Plato 360 BC* (New York: C. Scribner's Sons, 1871), 20.

Jung's Collective Consciousness and Synchronicity

Famed philosopher Carl Jung referred to anamnesis in his papers:

"Psychoanalysis is nothing but a somewhat deep and complicated form of anamnesis."[6]

Because another definition of anamnesis involves a medical patient who discloses their prior conditions, Jung seemed to be referring to that aspect of recollection rather than how it relates to reincarnation.

Jung also contributed other notable items worth discussing here, including his concept of the collective consciousness. One could argue that rather than tapping into our own past lives, we are simply tapping into memories from others who have lived throughout the ages.

Did we actually have the past lives we recalled during hypnosis, or are these memories simply far-flung examples of us tapping into the collective consciousness? This concept presupposes that all people share a collective memory of the past that is archetypal in nature and can be drawn upon through a shared memory. I believe in this wholeheartedly, and during sessions with clients, I sometimes intuitively feel they're tapping into the collective, rather than their own memories of their past lives. Still, this phenomenon is nothing like Supretrovie, which is experienced in waking consciousness and is often far more detailed and specific to the individual experience.

Lenz Theory of Enhanced Soul Awareness Through Meditation

In his book *Lifetimes*, the late Dr. Frederick Lenz explored self-induced spontaneous past life recall and described how this awareness could be enhanced through the practice of meditation and trance states without seeking assistance from a hypnotherapist. He described the uncanny feeling of familiarity you may feel with someone you have been with during a prior incarnation.

---

6. C. G. Jung, *Collected Papers on Analytical Psychology* (London: Balliere, Tindall and Cox, 1920), 206.

Lenz described that at times, simply meeting a person whom you knew in a prior incarnation could trigger memories of past lives. While I did not initially study those familiar encounters as part of my Supretrovie research, we will be exploring these cases in *Blast from the Past*, because these encounters can also cause the same phenomenon to occur. The difference between Supretrovie and what Dr. Lenz described is the fact that those who experience Supretrovie are not in any kind of trance or meditative state at all when these flashes happen. Clients reported gazing into the eyes of people they'd known before and simply having modern surroundings wash away.

Summing Up

Overall, there are a variety of reasons why a person may experience a flash of insight from a former life. Has it happened to you? Coming up, we will explore case histories of people bombarded by impressions from beyond their current life experience. Later, in part 3, you will have a chance to explore these possibilities for yourself.

PART ONE

· · · · · · · · ·

CASE STUDIES

ONCE I CONSCIOUSLY CAME to terms with what happened to me in Key West and how past life regression healed an issue I didn't even know I had, I began contemplating the implications that we are indeed more influenced by prior lifetimes than we may have ever thought before. I became convinced that things making people unbelievably unhappy could be remedied by recognizing the possibility for healing and going through the regression process to identify the true source event of the disturbance. This epiphany hit me like a ton of bricks. I felt elated, like I wanted to shout from the rooftops and tell others about Supretrovie in case they too had had terrible experiences that needed to be healed.

That's exactly what I did. In this next section, I will share some incredible case histories of clients who relayed both pleasant and unpleasant blasts from their pasts and found resolution by courageously facing these situations head-on through past life regression. Case histories are one of the most helpful parts of my book projects because when you're able to read about people who may be going through challenges similar to your own and who resolved those issues, you can walk away with hope that your own situation will indeed improve.

We will explore several kinds of Supretrovie in these studies, including those geographically induced from travel, artifacts, antiques and objects, gems and stones, and the irrefutable connections we have when meeting familiar people from our past. Supretrovie caused by traveling to familiar locations has remained my main focus for this research due to my personal experiences of being continually bombarded by emotional highs and lows during trips.

I hope you will find this information a helpful forerunner to part 3 of the book where you will have a chance to do some healing work of your own. For now, enjoy the stories, but most of all, be inspired. Life is filled with wonders as we traverse various ups and downs. Know that you can resolve deeply embedded challenges, and the following pages are filled with people who have done just that. Enjoy!

Chapter One

• • • •

GEOGRAPHICALLY INDUCED SUPRETROVIE

THE FACT THAT SO many people have similar experiences initially shocked me. In this chapter, we will explore fascinating examples of trips that yielded far more than memories and vacation photos in various places around the world.

Past Lives in Europe

One of my most dramatic Supretrovie experiences happened quite unexpectedly on another cruise from Barcelona to Rome. As usual, I felt spiritually called to Barcelona and had dreamed of going there for years. Once I arrived, I didn't love it as much as I'd hoped. Little did I know, I would soon be in for quite a surprise. On the way to Rome, we stopped in Naples, Italy. Travelers rave about Naples, but I never even thought of visiting there.

The morning the ship docked in the Port of Naples, I sat on the top deck, relaxing with a cup of coffee while watching the ship draw closer to the shore. That's when I saw something that took my breath away—a giant castle right on the shoreline. To my stunned amazement, the moment it came into full view, I began to cry uncontrollably. Fortunately, I hid myself from other passengers so they would not think I'd gone nuts. I sensed not only a place I loved, but a person I loved from times long gone.

The ship pulled into port, and I had a whole day of tours planned in Sorrento and Pompeii. I kept praying that we would make it back in time for me to go closer to the gargantuan structure. Fortunately, we did. That's both the blessing and curse of going on a cruise. The great news is you get to see a lot of things in a short period of time. The bad news is that it's a short period of time. If you hate a place, that's awesome! You'll soon be on your way. But if you love a place, well, you may be out of luck if you can't hurry around to see it all.

My friends were exhausted, so while they went back to the ship, I walked up to the castle. It was built in the 1200s. The closer I got, the more emotional I became. I stood by the wall and placed my hand on it, and somehow that helped a little. When the soul encounters something so emotional and familiar, that can be a real jolt to the system. You have to take a breath and get used to being there in the first place. Fortunately, that happened, and I spent several minutes basking in the awesome energy of the magnificent ramparts.

Soon though, I had to head back to the ship. I walked away, turning every so many feet so I could somehow say goodbye. I sensed more than ever a love story must have been involved.

Later that day, my friends and I were eating in the dining room. I felt the ship pull away from the dock, and I excused myself from the table and ran to the railing to watch while we left the port, sobbing quietly the whole time, just like a smitten schoolgirl.

Compelled to find out, I had a regression with some of my students and recalled my life as a young girl back in the 1200s who fell head over heels in love with the king who was already betrothed to another woman, so I loved him from afar. When I learned of his death at sea, my heart broke. I became inconsolable, although I could not tell anyone why.

What an emotional roller coaster! Naples is definitely a city in my heart and soul! I'd be curious to see how I would react going back there now that I've had the regression. I would expect those over-the-top emotions to taper off a bit. We shall see if I ever make it there again.

Likewise, this next section will explore other clients who had Supretrovie experiences in Europe. Enjoy!

Alysia Envisioned Her Former Home on a European Train

Alysia responded to the survey I sent out to find out who had strange experiences while traveling and relayed the following story:

"My parents loved Agatha Christie novels, and so I grew up with a sort of prebuilt fascination for the Orient Express, and I spent years daydreaming about taking it somewhere. My husband had business in London several years ago, and I went with him. Before we left, I did some research to see if we could ride the Orient Express. It's super expensive and really doesn't travel very long routes, so we decided to go on another line. After he finished all his meetings, we left London and took a train up north to York and then headed back to London, rode through the Channel Tunnel to Paris, then returned to London. My husband spent the extra money, so we were in first class and had a private car. It wasn't the Orient Express, but I loved it. Something odd happened during our final stretch between London and Paris. I looked out at the landscape, and I remember feeling a little dizzy. My husband thought I might have eaten something bad, but now that you mention it, I've always wondered if I had been there before. Something about that area sticks with me to this day. Not Paris or any of the bigger cities, but this tiny village we rode through somewhere in England. I would definitely be interested in finding out."

Alysia and I set up a session to find out more about her connection to England, train travel, and the Orient Express. Here's what happened:

SK: Where are you?

Alysia: I'm on a train.

SK: The Orient Express?

Alysia: Not necessarily, but it is nice. I have a private car and the space is very luxurious.

SK: Where are you and where are you going?

Alysia: I'm in London. I think I'm heading home.

SK: From where?

Alysia: A business trip comes to mind.

SK: Very good. What year is this?

Alysia: 1829.

SK: How do you feel?

Alysia: Not as excited as I thought I would be. I am very wealthy, so for me, this seems normal rather than special.

SK: Are you alone or with other people?

Alysia: My husband. He's there. He had business there and I went with him.

SK: Anyone else?

Alysia: No.

SK: How old are you?

Alysia: [Pausing] Late twenties maybe. We don't have any children.

SK: As you experience the energy of your husband in that lifetime, is he anyone you know in your current life?

Alysia: [After a moment] He may be a guy I dated for a short time in high school.

SK: What lessons did the two of you learn in that life and in this life?

Alysia: He only cared about money. Very materialistic in both lives. I did not want to continue with him this time around. I don't think we were very happy in the past, and I somehow knew that. I wanted a chance to experience a more down-to-earth existence with someone who knows how to show his feelings better.

SK: Very good. Go ahead and allow yourself to move through these experiences and arrive at your destination. Fast-forward to the next most significant event in your life in 1829 and notice what happens.

Alysia: Okay. I'm home.

SK: Where is your home?

Alysia: (Gasps) It's that little village! The one I saw on the train!

SK: Very good. What country is it in?

Alysia: Definitely England.

SK: Do you know the name?

Alysia: No. I had a flash of the White Cliffs of Dover. It's not far from there.

SK: Nice. What happens next?

Alysia: My husband is angry about storm damage that occurred while we were away. We own a large country estate. High winds damaged our barn, and some of our livestock escaped. He's yelling at a servant, angry he didn't do more.

SK: Imagine you can arrive at the very last day of your life. Be there now. Notice what's happening.

Alysia: I'm sick in bed. My husband is nowhere to be found. That same servant, the one he scolded, is there with me trying to help me.

SK: Is the servant anyone you know in your current life?

Alysia: My husband! He always stays with me, cares for me, and is by my side for all the ups and downs of life.

SK: What lessons did you learn in this life in England?

Alysia: Money means nothing without love. The husband there acted the same way in this current life. My then-boyfriend and I were at a movie theater once, and he became belligerent at someone who worked there. He shouted and made a horrible scene. I broke up with him over it and soon met my wonderful husband. I realize that while the extravagant things may be exciting to dream about, they mean nothing without true love. My husband stood by my side back then, and he's still there for me now. I made the right choice.

Do souls choose certain experiences before they arrive? Are we meant to meet certain people we've known before to replay things from our past? Do soul mates find a way to reunite throughout time? Alysia used her regression to deepen her commitment to her loving husband and knew at the experiential level that money can't buy love. I haven't heard from her since our session, but I do wish her and her husband well.

Simon's Illness Energetically Originated in Amsterdam

Simon came for a past life regression because he needed healing for a grave diagnosis—lung cancer. A nonsmoker his whole life, Simon's doctors did not give him a very positive prognosis for his future.

"I never smoked. Not ever. But now here I am, and they've said that even with treatment, I may not last another five years. I'm doing everything the doctors tell me—changing my diet, taking my treatments, but at this point, I'm open to anything and wanted to see if past life regression could help."

During the session, Simon expressed deep regret at not seeing his late grandfather before he died. That sadness and other heavy energy needed to move, so with the help of his guardian angel, Simon imagined releasing unwanted sadness and darker energies by placing them inside a trash can while a cosmic vacuum sucked tar and darkness from his lungs. We concentrated on moving healing light and high frequency transformational energy through his lungs once the darker colors dissipated. He envisioned himself as healthy and his lungs as bright, white, and in a state of perfect health.

Once we finished that part of the session, Simon delved into past lives. Up to that point, I had no clue we were about to uncover a Supretrovie, because he didn't bring up his trip to the Netherlands until we were already in the middle of his session, and I asked him to return to the source of his medical challenge. Simon soon realized his lung cancer had a definite connection with the past:

SK: Where are you?

Simon: Amsterdam.

SK: Very good. What year is this?

Simon: 1932.

SK: Very good. What's happening in Amsterdam in 1932?

Simon: I'm a man, older, overweight. I smoke nonstop. Smoking's a huge part of the culture. Now that I think of it, I visited there a few years ago, and nothing's changed. Man, did those people love to smoke! I remember during my vacation feeling that I'd been on the same streets at some point in the past. There's even a windmill off in the distance I remember seeing on my trip.

SK: What purpose did your soul have for living in Amsterdam?

Simon: To learn to experience joy through the simple things in life.

SK: Why did you choose to return there in your current life?

Simon: Because I really did love it there. My health wasn't the best, but I had lots of friends, lots to do, and the city was gorgeous.

SK: Was this your first life in Amsterdam?

Simon: No.

SK: Go back to the source of your connection. Be there now. What year is this?

Simon: 1774.

SK: Very good. Are you a man or a woman?

Simon: A man.

SK: How old are you?

Simon: Mid-twenties? Thirty, maybe.

SK: Describe your life there.

Simon: Busy. I am in the city. I enjoy the bustling of activity, the theater and entertainment. I had a good social life.

SK: Do you smoke?

Simon: Oh, yes—quite a bit. I drink a lot, too. We had a lot of beers in the pubs. Fun times.

SK: Very good. How old are you?

Simon: Maybe early thirties tops.

SK: Imagine you can fast-forward to the very last day of your life in 1700s Amsterdam. Notice how you pass into spirit.

Simon: Consumption.

SK: Very good. Go ahead and float into the peaceful space between lives. Be there now. What lessons did you learn in that life?

Simon: I didn't.

SK: Excuse me?

Simon: I didn't learn. I should know that you can't abuse the body. I wasn't even overweight. I was a tall, skinny kid who should have lived a long life, but I took stupid risks and trashed my body. That's why my life was cut short. You can't expect much else unless you take care of yourself.

SK: Imagine you are floating over the 1700s. Float forward in time so you are back at your life in 1900s Amsterdam. Be there now in an event that you most need to see at this moment. Notice what's happening.

Simon: I'm on the street. I'm struggling and can't breathe. I fall down. Somebody's coming, trying to help me, but I'm dying. I sense my lungs are black. They carry me someplace and put me in bed. They say I had a mini heart attack. They're giving me a drink of something to help: medicine of some kind. I'm in such bad health. I'm coughing.

SK: Do you recover?

Simon: I do.

SK: Fast-forward over time to the last day of your life in 1900s Amsterdam and be there now. How did you pass away during your second time in Amsterdam?

Simon: I'm back in the street again. After my earlier heart attack, I didn't even try to quit smoking or drinking. I'm out there again, but this time I had a bigger heart attack. I fell in the street. I hear people yelling for help. People gather around me, trying to comfort me, but I don't make it.

SK: Very good. Surrounded by a golden healing light, go ahead and lift again into the peaceful space between lives. What lessons did you learn in your second life in Amsterdam?

Simon: In that life, I was much older, like in my forties or fifties. I was out of shape and abused food, booze, and cigars. I didn't learn to take care of myself, and because of my age, I suffered in the end. I had a lot of great friends, but in the end, I learned nothing about my health. I did learn loyalty, though. I was a good friend to people who were close to me.

SK: And how were your two lives in Amsterdam similar?

Simon: Both of them were kind of the same. I wouldn't stop doing things I knew were no good for my health. The kid in the earlier life died easy. The older man struggled and suffered.

SK: How are these experiences affecting you in your current lifetime?

Simon: I somehow knew that I had to take care of myself, even from an early age. I never ever drank much. Even in school when all my buddies liked to party, I always said no. Yeah, they made fun of me, but I stuck to my convictions. I knew I couldn't do that. I also do my best not to overeat. I'll indulge on special occasions, but not very often. Still, it's discouraging to think what's happening to me now. It's like I can't get away from my health problems even when I try to do better.

SK: Why did your soul want to return to Amsterdam in this current lifetime?

Simon: Amsterdam is my favorite city on Earth, but looking back now, I wish I hadn't gone there. It seems like I picked up something bad there, like the energy followed me into this life. I didn't have any health problems at all until I came back from that trip.

SK: Did you pick up smoking on your trip to Amsterdam in your current life?

Simon: No. I remember seeing some people on the street smoking and thinking they looked relaxed. But no, I didn't partake. I never had in this life. The smoke swirled all around us, though. Everyone smokes. There's no avoiding secondhand smoke. They're good people, but in terms of health, they haven't changed much over the past couple hundred years.

SK: Were these lives in Amsterdam the true source events for your challenges with your lungs in your current lifetime?

Simon: Yes, absolutely.

SK: Are you ready to let this old energy go?

Simon: Yes, 100 percent.

Is it possible for an illness to come through into your life simply by returning to the source of a past life problem? Simon certainly believed so. We did a cord cutting and worked to heal the energy and disconnect the residual energies from his past and present. Simon made an agreement with his soul and Higher Self that he no longer needed to be influenced by the energy of those former lives. He acknowledged that he made conscious choices to be not only a loyal friend to others in his current lifetime, but to take better care of his health.

While I am not sure if this regression will help him in the distant future, I last heard from Simon a few years into his diagnosis, and his condition had not worsened. He had implemented a strict dietary plan that included proper foods, plenty of rest, and exercise. His doctors revised their initial projection for his life expectancy and told him he had a chance to recover by continuing with his new diet and health regimen.

Bernice Discovered Prehistoric Roots

I always enjoy talking about travel with anyone who wants to share their vacation experiences with me, and I wound up getting into a conversation with Bernice, whom I met at one of my seminars. Somehow, we got talking about cruises in the Mediterranean and the fascinating port of Gibraltar, which these days is partly controlled by both the UK and Spain. Gibraltar is a quirky place. The strategic location made it an important territory for military powers even during the times of Napoleon. At the same time, the famed Rock of Gibraltar remains a historic geological wonder, in addition to several amazing cave complexes. I mentioned my trip to the Saint Michael's Cave, filled with stunning limestone stalagmites, and she described a boat ride to another historic site:

"The moment the ship docked and I walked on the ground there, I felt a powerful, grounded feeling. We took a boat trip out to Gorham's Cave, and when I glanced inside, my body disappeared, and everything became quiet for a moment. I don't know why that happened, but I did like the area."

Bernice decided to find out more about the experience by going on a past life regression. At first, I assumed she must have been some former naval commander or a member of an ancient army. The historical possibilities were endless in such a colorful location. To my surprise and hers, she'd been in the area much earlier than any of those conflicts:

SK: Go back to the source event of your connection with the area we know as Gibraltar. Be there now. Notice what's happening. What year is this?

Bernice: So early.

SK: Are you a man or woman?

Bernice: A man.

SK: Are you alone or with other people?

Bernice: I'm with a small group. We're carving tools, trying to spear fish and survive.

SK: Do you have a family?

Bernice: No, not how we would think of family today. This is prehistoric. We don't have anything but our stone and bone tools. We wear skins for clothing. We make sounds, but don't have language. We climb and live in the caves and use the caves for protection from the elements and other predators.

SK: Go to the last day of your life. Be there now. Notice how you pass into spirit.

Bernice: I'm injured from a fall off a high cliff. I chased a bird, tried to catch it, and my foot slipped. I fell and hit myself against the jagged rocks and fell into the ocean. I might have been able to swim, but my injuries were too severe, so I drowned.

SK: Float into the peaceful space between lives. Be there now. What lessons did you learn in that early time?

Bernice: To survive the best I can.

SK: Why did your soul choose to return to that place in your current life as Bernice?

Bernice: To remember the land. To remember how to live simply and to be grateful for everything I have and to live moment by moment without expectation.

As it turns out, the Gibraltar area and Gorham's Cave Complex held evidence that Neanderthals lived in that area thousands of years ago, long before recorded history.[7] Could Bernice have lived in those incredibly early times? It's certainly possible. Thanks to the wonders of carbon dating and advances in archaeology, we're learning that humankind is far older and more advanced than we ever imagined.

Madeline Recalled Her Past Life in the Icy North

Earlier, I mentioned that I am a big cruise lover, probably thanks to my past lives at sea. What I've found over the years is that those who enjoy cruising were also likely replaying the things they loved and enjoyed in past lives, and Madeline definitely fit that description. I've found that all people who love cruising tend to enjoy sharing stories, so I was enthralled to hear Madeline's story about her adventures at sea.

---

7. World Heritage List, "Gorham's Cave Complex," *Unesco*, 2016, https://whc.unesco.org/en /list/1500/.

Madeline became a travel agent specializing in cruising back in the days before cruises were as affordable or popular as they are now. She relayed an interesting story about a *hallucination*, as she called it, during her trip to Northern Europe that she didn't quite know what to make of:

"I stood out on deck early one morning on the front of the ship, watching the ice crack into the sea just off the coast of Norway, and I happened to look out a ways toward a mountainous area when I saw a cabin appear in my mind's eye, with smoke coming out the chimney. I had a feeling of standing in heavy clothes in the snow with a fur-lined hood around my face. A moment later, I came back to the present day. My friends always said I'm a creative type, but this seemed like something beyond my imagination."

Madeline decided to have a regression to uncover why she loved cruising and Norway in particular:

SK: What year is this?

Madeline: 1713.

SK: Where are you?

Madeline: Norway, in a cabin deep in the woods near that same area I saw in my mind.

SK: Are you alone or with others?

Madeline: I am a man and I have a wife and a few children. We're in the cabin, and my wife is cooking. The kids are playing. It's a very difficult existence, fighting with nature and the cold, but it's also a good life.

SK: What lessons did you learn there?

Madeline: Simplicity.

SK: How are you applying that lesson in your current life?

Madeline: [Chuckling] I'm not. I wish I could. Life was hard back then, but in a way, things were also simpler. Being outdoors, quiet, and knowing what matters in life are things I wish I could enjoy more.

I think that's why I love being a travel agent, though, because I help people get outside and enjoy things that are beyond the daily pressures of life.

SK: Does this explain your love of cruising?

Madeline: No.

SK: Go back to the source event where you first came to love the sea. Be there now. Where are you?

Madeline: I'm from England, but at the moment, I'm on a ship bound for Africa.

SK: What year is this?

Madeline: 1549?

SK: What's happening?

Madeline: I am a deckhand. Very young. Hard worker. This is the best job I can get that pays well, and despite the hard conditions, I feel free in the sea. I stand on the ship and enjoy the wind blowing in my face. I can't stand around long, but every so often, I'm able to enjoy it, and I love the feeling of freedom.

A free spirit during her current lifetime, Madeline certainly did help people. She's since passed away and is sorely missed. I'm sure her clients are forever grateful to her for introducing them to cruising, because it's an experience that seems to resonate with so many who I believe had past lives at sea. Returning to those familiar experiences is healing for the soul.

Past Lives in Asia

Asia has become one of my personal favorite travel destinations in recent years. Another strong Supretrovie experience happened during my Christmastime trip to Japan. When I arrived in Tokyo, I stayed in the famous Shinjuku neighborhood at the luxurious Park Hyatt Hotel. One of the main tourist attractions is the Tokyo Metropolitan Government Building observation deck that stands 202 meters high and gives outstanding views of the city. After a grueling flight, my friend and I dropped our stuff off at the hotel and headed straight to that tower. I will never forget the moment I stood in that building and first glimpsed the glittering night skyline of Tokyo. I cried. I couldn't stop. Not from sorrow, but from joy. I remember a distinct feeling of not recognizing a single bit of the gorgeous city below, but the beautiful land called me, and a deep sense of *thank God I'm finally home* came over me. I had a little movie run in my mind of a flatter area with few structures in a time hundreds, if not thousands, of years ago.

My love didn't stop with Tokyo. The funny thing about any travel is that typically the places I've loved the most were ones I had never thought of visiting before. After purchasing a rail pass and traveling for a week all over this stunning country, a last-second decision landed me in the spectacular Nagano, home of the 1998 Winter Olympics.

I stopped in the Nagano station with the intention of going out to see the amazing snow monkeys who live in hot springs in that area, but by the time I arrived, the tours had all gone out for the day. With no plan, my friend and I decided to take a stroll through the town to go visit one of the many Buddhist temples that are plentiful throughout Japan.

Nagano is stunning. The alpine setting and wood buildings give you a sense of a true winter village, especially since the temperatures plummeted below freezing. Frigid air encouraged me to walk a little faster to try to stay warm. That magnetic pull toward the temple only increased as I walked through those streets and began to experience another feeling of deep love drawing me in toward the site.

We stopped in a tourist booth to speak to the staff and pick up a map and temple information when I felt suddenly overcome with emotion and had to literally bite my lip to keep from crying. With the Zenkoji Temple in sight, I once again felt like I had finally arrived at my beloved home, and the joyful feeling nearly overcame me. The staff explained the current structure had only been around for a few hundred years because the temple had burned to the ground a few different times over the centuries.

I felt no connection to the actual building, but to the land itself. Like Tokyo, I realized the place itself without anything modern drew me in, and the immense gratitude I felt and still feel at having had a chance to go there is something that makes me emotional even now. I pulled out some of my souvenir pamphlets from the area to glance at while writing this section, and tears filled my eyes yet again.

I'm currently in the middle of teaching a past life regression certification course, so I asked one of my students to regress me to Nagano for this book. I discovered my life as a monk in ancient times. I could not give a date, but I saw myself outside in a ceremony where a master poured water over my head. Outside the Zenkoji Temple today is a wonderful fountain with blessed water, and I partook in washing my face and hands in this life as well, which brought great emotion. During the regression, I could see why, even though this time around, I did not have any masters assisting me.

A second vision of Zenkoji involved me sitting in a temple with hundreds of other monks. Far in the back of the crowded room, I sensed my days filled with a steady combination of silence and chanting. Overall, the life felt like pure joy.

Back in 2019, over my birthday weekend, I had a unique opportunity to stay at a Buddhist temple for a ten-day silent retreat that changed my life and brought back deep memories of lives like the one I lived in Japan. I recognized the friend who steered me toward the temple in my current life had also been with me in Japan long ago. Not surprising. To this day, I can still say, of all the places in the world that I love with all my heart, Japan is close to the top, if not at the very top, of my list of favorite places. I could say that I recommend you go there, too, but I know that while one person loves a place, another person may have a totally different experience. This is thanks to our individuality and karma from the past. Still, if something calls to you about this place or any of the places in this book, you may want to pay a visit yourself sometime.

Like me, the following clients also had interesting stories to share from trips around Asia, and they likewise found healing and understanding about unusual thoughts that occurred to them while exploring this incredible part of our world.

Candice Connected with her Cambodian Roots

Candice and I began talking about Asia, and she told me all about her visit to Cambodia, a place I would still like to visit in the future. She'd been daydreaming about visiting the holy temples in Angkor Wat for a couple of decades, ever since she first saw the area featured on television:

"I grew up in rural Nebraska, raised by a very conservative family, so I know there's no way I had any preconceptions about what I might find in a place like Cambodia. I'm not even sure I ever gave that country a single thought in my entire life until I saw that show on TV. The second I saw those temples, my brain buzzed. I became obsessed with finding out every little thing about the place. As I've gotten older, I have been on my own journey away from the religious upbringing I had on our family farm. My parents were strict Christians. To think I had such strong feelings about such a remote part of the world is unheard of, and yet, I could not get it out of my mind. I started looking into Buddhism, and for years, I've always had some kind of inner knowing that I must have lived there in a past life. I think I may have been one of the monks. I searched around for trips and found a spiritual group offering a tour there, so I saved up and went. The people there are amazing, and the sites are beautiful. A peaceful feeling overwhelmed me at times. I felt like I'd come home."

Candice found the answers she received during her regression were not what she expected.

SK: Where are you?

Candice: In a small hut in a jungle.

SK: What part of the world?

Candice: It's there. Cambodia, near the temples.

SK: Very good. What year is it?

Candice: I'm not sure. Early.

SK: What were you doing during your life in Cambodia?

Candice: I'm a little girl. I live in a tiny home with my family and brothers. We are poor but happy. My oldest brother is about to go away to become a monk. My parents are very proud and happy for him.

SK: What is your connection with Angkor Wat?

Candice: The temple area is a place our family visits. Once my brother becomes a monk, he makes journeys to Angkor Wat, but he lives in another area.

SK: Fast-forward through your life to the next most significant event. Be there now.

Candice: I am still home with my parents, tending to people near our home.

SK: Do you ever serve as a monk yourself?

Candice: No, but I do serve the monks and others in the community. I help feed and care for them when they're sick. I am like a nurse. A caregiver.

SK: How does that life relate to your current lifetime?

Candice: Although I wasn't an actual monk, I learned about peacefulness there, and also, I still work in healthcare. I'm a nurse practitioner. I am so happy we have all the advancements in medicine these days that we obviously didn't have way back then, but what's just as important is love and caring for people. Love heals.

Candice discovered her purpose had deeper roots than she imagined and gained insight into her life journey, and although she didn't find what she expected, the understanding of her commitment to care for others brought her a deeper sense of peace and self-understanding. I've seen

Candice a few times since our session, and she continues to do well as a member of the healthcare community.

Otis Experienced a Jolt on a Thai Trip

I met Otis at a metaphysical expo. He had long been interested in past life regression even though he had never had one, and somehow we began discussing travel, and he told me about something that happened to him years earlier during his backpacking adventure in Thailand:

"Bangkok was wild. I knew I had been there before after spending several nights in different hotels. We wound up taking a train out of town, and a sick feeling really hit me when we passed through a small village and went over the River Kwai. I remember looking out the window and feeling ill. I got over it once we were back out in the countryside, but I've always wondered about that. I think I was one of the workers who built the bridge in World War II."

At first, Otis seemed to have had an anamnesis about his former life in Thailand. The soul often recalls such past experiences, but in Otis's case, he was in for a huge surprise. Here's what happened:

SK: Go ahead and travel back into the past to a time that would most explain your familiar feeling in Thailand. Be there now. Notice what's happening. What year is this?

Otis: 1942.

SK: Very good. Where are you?

Otis: Thailand.

SK: Very good. Notice what's happening.

Otis: [After a moment] I'm outside.

SK: Are you alone or with other people?

Otis: I'm alone at the moment, but other people are nearby.

SK: How do you feel?

Otis: Angry.

SK: Why do you feel angry?

Otis: I'm supervising construction, and these workers are not going fast enough. If they don't do better, I could be put to death.

SK: Fast-forward through these events. See what happens next.

Otis: There are so many dying. They're hungry; they're sick.

SK: How does that make you feel?

Otis: Terrible, but I still have a job to do, and the structure is so messed up. Many people aren't going to make it.

SK: Fast-forward to the last day of your life. Be there now. How do you pass into spirit?

Otis: I'm sick.

SK: What year is that?

Otis: 1943 comes to mind.

SK: Very good. How does this lifetime relate to your current life?

Otis: I've had some really hard times at work in the past. That's my karma. I had to meet certain people this time and repay the debt by allowing them to mistreat me. I've had coworkers steal from me; I've had car wrecks. You name it. Things are better now, but for a while, my life felt chaotic.

SK: Have you paid that debt now?

Otis: Yes.

SK: Very nice. What else have you done to repay this debt? Couldn't there be another way for you to pay your debt other than having others mistreat you?

Otis: Yes. I do other things like volunteering, helping people who don't have access to good food or proper healthcare. I'm on the board of our local homeless shelter. I'm trying to do better now.

SK: Why did you return to Thailand in your current life?

Otis: I had to go see that. It's helping me somehow. I can never, ever in this life, or even if I have other lives after this one—I can never do anything like that again. It would be better to die honorably than to feel forced into mistreating people. I won't make that mistake again.

Once in a while, I run into people fascinated by certain times in history who are convinced they lived a certain way, only to realize that they played the exact opposite role. Otis had indeed described the Thai Death Bridge built by the Japanese in World War II to facilitate their passage to Burma. Considered a human rights catastrophe, the bridge project caused thousands to perish from illness and accidents.[8] Otis seemed to have truly evolved as a soul since then and has become a pillar of his community. There's always room for improvement in the soul journey.

Summing Up

The soul is so vast, it makes sense that various places we've lived before engender either incredibly positive or negative feelings when we visit. Hopefully these clients' stories gave you pause to reconsider some of your own trips in the past that you either loved or hated. Perhaps now, you, too, may find yourself asking, "Did I live there before?" The answer to that question may provide startling insights into the depths of your soul.

---

8. Chris Wotton, "Death Railway: History of the Bridge on the River Kwai," *The Culture Trip*, July 17, 2018, https://theculturetrip.com/asia/thailand/articles/bridge-on-the-river-kwai-a -place-to-remember-thailands-past/.

Chapter Two

• • • •

SUPRETROVIE FROM ARTIFACTS & OBJECTS

WHENEVER I TRAVEL, I love to pick up local crafts from the artisans in the markets who are out trying to make a living. I have a real soft place in my heart for these amazing entrepreneurs, and at one time, I'd amassed quite a collection of oddities. As I travel down the road of life, I am getting less and less materialistic and find having too many belongings to be a real energetic distraction. To remedy this, I began selling off my treasures at metaphysical shows.

One of my favorite hobbies that's come out of this is watching people gravitate to things at my table. You can really tell a lot about a person and, from my perspective, a lot about their past lives by watching the things that attract them. These art sales have generated a lot of fun conversations through the years that led to discovering the prevalence of our connection to objects. Cherished objects can indeed carry the energy from prior owners into the awareness of unsuspecting people, but can they also ignite deeply embedded memories from times long gone? I say yes, absolutely!

We will also discuss what happens when people encounter ancient artifacts in museum settings, which can really send people into strong Supretrovie situations. Years ago, I visited the Kremlin Armory Museum in Moscow as an excursion during a Russian Volga River cruise and ran straight into a carriage I know I had been in close proximity to in a prior lifetime. The force of this recollection nearly knocked me off my feet. To date, that's still my strongest example of artifact-induced Supretrovie, but the clients you'll read about in this section experienced all kinds of freaky phenomena from various artifacts and objects that led them to make a powerful past life connection.

Tyrone Recalled His Death by Touching a Jamaican Tomb

No doubt there can be super spooky vibes and creepy happenings around gravesites. Tyrone discovered this firsthand when he went with friends to the lovely island of Jamaica. His friends persuaded him to go on a tour of one of the most famous landmarks on the island where he picked up weird vibes near the tomb of one of the island's most notorious residents:

"My friends wanted to take tours, which I wasn't so excited about because I wanted to sit on the beach, but I went along with them anyway. We took a bus through the jungle and up to the top of this hill that overlooked the ocean to the old mansion where this lady known as the White Witch lived. The place looked incredible, and the views were great, but I felt really ill there, especially after they offered us some rum punch right at the end of the tour. We were gathered around outside, and I accidentally brushed up against the stone coffin of the lady who owned the place. Right after that, I started heaving and getting sick. I never even considered a past life connection, though. I assumed I was overheated because we'd been drinking a little too much."

I had also been to the Rose Hall, home of the famed White Witch who had supposedly murdered several of her spouses and now haunted the residence,[9] so Tyrone's story fascinated me, and I wanted to know more. His regression revealed he had a close tie to the mysterious estate:

SK: Return to the source event of your connection with Rose Hall in Jamaica. Be there now. Notice what's happening.

Tyrone: I am in a living room.

SK: Very good. Are you a man or woman?

Tyrone: A man.

SK: Are you with other people or alone?

Tyrone: I'm with my wife.

SK: How do you feel?

Tyrone: Happy.

SK: Fast-forward through the events of your life in Jamaica. Notice if there are any major conflicts there.

Tyrone: Troubles with crops, an occasional illness, but no. Nothing terrible.

SK: Fast-forward to the last day of your life. Be there now. Notice how you pass away.

Tyrone: I catch a flu or some illness. I have a high fever and drift away, my wife by my side.

SK: As you float now into the peaceful space between lives, do you sense any ill will your wife held toward you during your experience in Jamaica?

---

9. Herbert G. De Lisser, *The White Witch of Rose Hall* (New York: Macmillan Education, 1929, 1982).

Tyrone: None at all. She seems like a wonderful person: very giving and generous. She always helped the neighbors and the people who worked there.

Despite the popularity of the story about the White Witch of Rose Hall, skeptics say the entire story about the haunting is a fabrication. Annie Palmer, the real woman who lived there and is said to haunt the estate, had four husbands, but she would never hurt a fly. Could it be that Tyrone was one of those fortunate men married to this kind soul? We can only speculate, but he definitely convinced me that his connection to the manor was very much a part of reality.

Wooden Carving Helped Callie Recall a Brief Life in Vietnam

Callie, a sweet girl in her twenties, purchased some of the handmade art I'd collected in different places around the world when we met at an expo. She immediately gravitated to a hand-carved wooden figure of a lady in a skirt complete with a traditional Vietnamese hat.

"I know where you got this," she giggled. "I went to Vietnam a couple of years ago. My grandpa fought over there, so my family didn't want me to go, but I went anyway. I love the people there and I felt so at home."

Through a regression, Callie recalled some other surprising details about her trip she hadn't initially remembered:

SK: Where are you and what year is this?

Callie: Vietnam, 1962.

SK: Very good. What's happening?

Callie: I am a little girl.

SK: Nice. How old are you?

Callie: Five.

SK: Who is with you in this lifetime?

Callie: I live in a house with my parents, brothers, sisters … maybe grandma and grandpa.

SK: Very good. How do you feel?

Callie: Scared. There is something bad happening. Fighting all the time. Pollution is horrible. People are getting sick.

SK: Protected by a healing light, float to the very last day of your life in Vietnam in the 1960s. Be there now. Notice how you pass into spirit.

Callie: Not too much later. There's war and explosions. I am hit, but I don't realize it's coming, so I do not suffer. I saw lots of people die before I did, though, so I struggled through the trauma of seeing my family getting sick and hurt.

SK: Float up, up, up, into that peaceful space between lives. Be there now. What lessons did you learn in that life in Vietnam?

Callie: Nothing matters but family.

SK: Why did your soul want to return to that place in your current life?

Callie: I loved the people there, and I still do. They did not deserve what happened to them. Oh, and I thought about something else. I remember I felt ill all of a sudden during my vacation and had a vision in my mind of smoke in the air. I think I picked up on something that happened during the war. It was scary. I hate what happened to the people there, but it's still a lovely place, and I am grateful to have had the chance to go back.

SK: How does this lifetime relate to your soul purpose?

Callie: I am a peace crusader. I have a full awareness that war and violent conflict are never the right answer.

Callie inspired me, and I feel confident as she moves through her life journey that she will carry that lesson with her to make the world a better place.

Violin Inspired Miles's Love of Music

Miles wanted to explore his past lives for curiosity's sake, which is quite common among my clients. He suggested several places he wanted to know about, including Egypt and Greece, because of his fascination with those parts of the world. Then he mentioned something striking that happened to him in childhood:

"My great-great grandmother played a violin. I never knew her because she passed away before I was born. When I was about five, my parents took me to my grandparents' house to stay one afternoon while they attended an event, and my grandmother pulled out my great-great grandmother's old violin and let me pluck the strings. From that moment on, I was obsessed. I can't say this falls into your spontaneous past life category or not, but I do know that everyone wondered why I knew how to play so well, even before I had lessons. Since then, I've been a semiprofessional musician. I've played for the local symphony and traveled overseas to perform in Europe. I've always wondered about my real attraction to music. I understand we're influenced by our family, but still, there must be more to it than just a family connection."

Miles's insight proved correct. Although new evidence suggests our personalities may be up to 20 percent influenced by our ancestral genes, Miles not only had his lineage on his side when it came to his musical talents, but past life memories as well. Here's what happened:

SK: Return to the source event where your soul first came to love the violin. Where are you? What year is it?

Miles: Late 1800s. Germany comes to mind.

SK: Very good. Are you a man or woman?

Miles: A man.

SK: What's happening there in 1800s Germany?

Miles: I'm a musician playing my violin with an orchestra in a ballroom.

SK: Nice. How do you feel?

Miles: [After a moment] Sad.

SK: What caused you to feel sad?

Miles: I enjoy the music and making people happy, but something happened, and I feel terrible. I don't want to be there playing. I want to be somewhere else.

SK: Imagine you can rewind and go back to the source event of your sadness. Be there now. Notice what's happening.

Miles: I'm in a bedroom. My mother is in the bed and she's dying.

SK: What happened to her?

Miles: Old age. She's caught a cold or something, and it just wore her down to the point of no return. There's a doctor there who says there's nothing anyone can do for her. I hate hearing that, but now I have to go work.

SK: Be back in the ballroom now, playing your violin. From there, fast-forward to the next most significant event in that life. Be there now. Where are you?

Miles: My mother's funeral. I'm standing outside in the frigid air; wind is whipping all around. We're looking into the grave.

SK: As you experience the energy of the people there, who is with you?

Miles: Family. Seems like a brother and some more distant relations. Our father already passed away.

SK: As you experience the energy of your mother, brother, and the other people gathered for the funeral, is there anyone you know in your current life?

Miles: [Gasps] Yes, my mother. She's my great-great grandmother. It's her.

SK: Good job. What lessons did the two of you come to learn together?

Miles: Music. My mother in Germany inspired my music. In my current life, even though she already passed on, finding my great-great grandmother's violin inspired me again in this life. It's like she left that violin there for me to find.

SK: How does music play into your soul's purpose?

Miles: Music is a big part of my purpose. To help others enjoy themselves and relax through music.

Once the session ended, I asked Miles if he had ever been to Germany, and he said that yes, he had traveled there during his time in Europe, but like many of my clients, he didn't recall any thoughts about being there in a prior lifetime. Many of us have impressions that seem so impossible, we instantly dismiss them, and then they cannot be retrieved in memory. For Miles, the object rather than the place brought his past lives to the forefront of his experience.

No doubt we're meant to be with certain people, especially our family and close friends, and in Miles's case, even though his great-great grandmother missed seeing him during his current life experience, she left him a gift that changed the course of his life and helped him fulfill his mission and purpose. I haven't seen Miles since, but I feel confident he's continuing to spread the joy of music to everyone he meets.

Elena Became Spellbound by a Croatian Cross

Like many of my clients, Elena had relationship problems that led her to seek a regression. Relationships come in all forms. In her mid-twenties, Elena struggled with challenging dynamics and trying to fit in with a domineering roommate who, according to her, sought to control every facet of daily life for her and the other girl who shared their apartment. During our talk before the session began, I talked about my Supretrovie research, and as a side note, Elena told me about a surprise when she received a beautiful souvenir from her aunt.

"My aunt, my mom's sister, went on a trip to Croatia a few years ago. We've always been very close since she doesn't have any kids of her own. I'm like a daughter to her. Still, I don't expect her to buy me anything when she goes on vacation. After she came home, she gave me a gorgeous gold cross. I couldn't believe the feeling I had when she first handed it to me. My whole body buzzed and got very warm. My mom thought I had the flu or something, but I swear I didn't. When I held the cross, I saw a beach and felt wind blowing my hair. I've never had anything like that happen before or since. I didn't want to tell my aunt or my mom what I saw or how I felt like I had been spiritually transported to some other time. They're both such devoted Catholics, I didn't want to scare them. I forgot all about it until you mentioned spontaneous memories. I'm not sure if this qualifies or not. I can't describe why that happened, or how, but I've always wondered about it."

Did Elena pick up on the vibrations of Croatia and the former Yugoslavia, or did she experience a residual residue from one of her own past lives in that region? We both wanted to find out, so she agreed to have a session. Little did we know the memory had much to do with the reason she sought the regression in the first place. Here's what we discovered:

SK: Return to the source event of your fascination with your cross. Be there now. Notice what's going on. Where are you?

Elena: I am in a church.

SK: Are you a man or woman?

Elena: Woman. I'm a nun.

SK: What year is this?

Elena: 1200s.

SK: Very good. How do you feel?

Elena: Peaceful. The life is hard, the conditions are terrible, but I have a good life compared to most. I spend most of my time preparing food for the poor, praying, tending to the sick.

SK: Rewind to the time before you entered this convent. How did you become a nun?

Elena: I married a man from the village at a very young age. He worked hard but acted abusive toward me, and shortly after we married, he died in an accident. My family banished me to the convent. That seems harsh, but I enjoyed the convent and found that life to be so much better than what I would have had if my husband had lived. I enjoyed the peace and quiet and praying.

SK: As you experience the energy of your family and your husband in that life, do any of them feel familiar?

Elena: [Gasps] It's her! My roommate.

SK: Which one?

Elena: [After a moment] I think they're both there in the convent with me. That's unreal!

SK: How did the life you had then relate to the life you have now?

Elena: The one who's giving us the problem had a higher ranking in the order than we did, like a headmistress or something. She liked to keep everything in its place, just so. She's still such a controlling person. She's always picking on me, trying to find fault with everything I do and singling me out from the others. She makes me scrub floors two or three times. I didn't get it, but now I see she hasn't changed much since then. When she passed away in our first life together, myself and several other nuns all felt like we'd been freed. We still had a hard life there for the times. The extremely cold, harsh conditions were tough to take, but we managed to find peace.

SK: What about your other roommate?

Elena: She never attacked my other roommate for some reason. She targeted me and some of the other nuns. Even my other roommate thought things improved after her death, though.

SK: What lessons are the three of you learning together in these lifetimes?

Elena: I found out that through prayer and silence, you can find happiness by connecting yourself with God. In this life, that can happen, too, but only if I send light to her and find my own quiet place within. I can't change her. I can only change myself. I know I could move, but none of us can afford that right now, so we're going to need to work it out somehow.

SK: How did the cross you received from your aunt relate to your life as a nun? Or did it?

Elena: The gold is familiar because it comes from that same area. My aunt must have tuned in to the idea that I needed that cross in my life to remind me to always remain thankful and to find my own happiness.

SK: Nice. Anything else?

Elena: I need to always remember that no matter how bad I may feel, others have a far more difficult path than I do.

We did a healing with her and her two roommates and the nuns to release any residual energy and disengage from the past. No doubt, despite the tumultuous past of the former Yugoslavia region, there are plenty of monasteries and convents all throughout modern Croatia with rich histories. I don't doubt that Elena tapped into a past life memory, and the gift she received from her aunt served as a reminder for her soul and a sign on her path to peace. I spoke to her after our session, and she said that the troubles with her roommate had significantly decreased since our session. All the girls were managing far better than before, which was great to hear. Like Elena, consider the possibility that true happiness is first created within the self. Gratitude and humbleness don't hurt, either. Elena had a bit of both, which I believe contributed to her success in overcoming this obstacle.

Linus Discovered His Former Home

Shortly before his wedding, Linus decided to have a past life regression to see if he and his soon-to-be wife were as connected as he thought. He said they'd been together forever, and after reading books on reincarnation, he started to believe that they'd been with each other in former lives. His story of their vacation brought that feeling to the forefront of his mind.

"My girlfriend and I recently graduated from college. To celebrate, I decided we should go overseas and take a long trip together—something we hadn't had a chance to do before now, and I planned to propose while we were there. We get along well and have a lot in common. Both of us have been fascinated by the idea of going to Spain after watching some shows and talking to mutual friends who have been over there. We did all the research to do the trip right and bought new backpacks and rail passes. She also wanted to see Paris, so we flew there, and I hoped to propose on the Eiffel Tower. We did the Paris thing first, and the engagement went well. I had it all planned out. I got on one knee right on the observation deck. She loved it. Then we went to Barcelona. Neither of us could get over the gorgeous scenery from the train. One day, we stopped at a tiny village along the route somewhere in the middle of nowhere in Northern Spain. We thought the place looked nice, so we decided to get off the train and wander around the countryside. We walked up to an abandoned farmhouse, and my new fiancée wanted to check it out. I wasn't sure at first, but she talked me into it. The inside had a bunch of rusted artifacts and one of those old metal irons that they would heat up on the fire in the old days. She picked it up and handed it to me. The second I touched it, I got transported back in time. I saw myself there, looking out at the Pyrenees Mountains. I felt like some enemy was watching me and that maybe I would die soon. It felt like two people in the same body—the mountain man and myself. I had a vision of being alone there and having my family die, and I sensed that for some reason I lived through whatever killed them. We couldn't find a place to stay in that town, so we got back on the train and went to Barcelona. That night in the hotel, I had a dream about that farmhouse. I dreamed my fiancée and I were there. I told her about it, but she didn't think it meant anything. She's always considered me to be a bit out-there. I do wonder what it meant, though."

Linus believed he made it all up, but soon he would discover that the soul really does return to familiar places from the past:

SK: What year is this?

Linus: 1639 comes to mind.

SK: What's happening?

Linus: This sounds insane, but I'm there in that house, only it's nice and newer. I am a farmer. There's a group stealing sheep and killing them, killing any people who stand in their way. They've been terrorizing the neighboring towns, and I know they're coming for me and my family next.

SK: As you experience the energy of your family and the other people living at that time, is there anyone who feels familiar to you?

Linus: Yes, she's there with me: my fiancée.

SK: Anyone else seem familiar?

Linus: No. We have two small children, both under the age of five, I'd say, but I don't know either of them.

SK: Fast-forward through that life and notice what happens next.

Linus: Thieves are coming. They're burning things, trying to take my livestock and anything else they can get their hands on. They try to kill us, but I put up a fight. I saved my family, but I'm injured, and I don't make it.

SK: What lessons did you learn in that lifetime that you're experiencing now?

Linus: Family is first; things don't matter at all.

After doing some healing around the trauma of their past life in Spain, Linus said he felt better. He also said the experience deepened his connection to his fiancée, and he knew more than ever that they were meant to be together as soul mates. Their wedding took place a few months after his session. I haven't heard from him since, but I wish them a current lifetime of happiness.

Georgia Connected to a Palatial Life Through an Antique Ring

Eccentric antique-dealing Georgia also worked as a part-time auctioneer and novice tarot reader. When she took an old garnet ring in on consignment from one of her steady customers, she experienced the unexpected:

"Normally I handle a lot of the consignments for our store, but one day while I was out, another employee took an old garnet ring into inventory and showed it to me when I returned to work. I do a little tarot on the side, and I'm fairly intuitive. I do pick up on energy from past owners of many of the items we carry. Normally I don't get too attached, though, because we have so many interesting antiques and oddities coming through the store. This situation shocked me. When the other employee handed that ring to me, I had a vision of an old-fashioned parlor, with jazz music playing in the background. I've held other objects in the past that made my fingers hurt, and that always lets me know I should cleanse those, but this time, I felt pulled into that energy. I had never had such a visual experience of anything from the store before. I do a lot of research about designs on glassware and jewelry and all that so I can learn about the items historically. That kind of detail helps sales, so I tried to find out anything I could about the ring, and when the other employee didn't know, I actually called the man who brought it in. He told me he received it as part of an inheritance after his aunt passed away. His wife had no interest in keeping it, so they decided to sell. I kept the ring in inventory for a couple of days. At night, I dreamt about it, and I couldn't stand the thought of anyone else buying it, so before the end of the week, I pulled it out of the auction and bought it myself. I've never had such a reaction before or since. I would love to know why."

Objects clearly carry vibrations and residual energy from those who owned them before. Psychometry is the art of picking up information from objects. You'll have a chance to do this yourself in the second half of the book. People who practice psychometry do so willingly with intention. Sensitive people like Georgia often pick up vibrations from items without even trying. She clearly mentioned recognizing when items needed to be cleared of unwanted influences, which told me that she indeed possessed the psychic gift of clairsentience, or knowing by feeling. Georgia's weird experience could have been a mere reflection of her obvious intuitive talents, or there could be more to the story. Psychometry can definitely be a trigger for Supretrovie. Could the owner return to the object in a later lifetime? Georgia and I were about to find out.

SK: Go back to the source event of your attraction to this garnet ring. Be there now. Notice what's happening.

Georgia: I'm in Hungary.

SK: Very good. What's going on in Hungary?

Georgia: I am a young woman in her late teens. I'm all dressed up and riding in a coach with two older women.

SK: Very good. As you experience the energy of these women, notice their relationship to you.

Georgia: They're my mother and grandmother. I am the only child, and my father passed away.

SK: Are either of them anyone you know in your current lifetime?

Georgia: No.

SK: Imagine you can fast-forward through these events and arrive at your destination. Notice what happens next.

Georgia: We have pulled up on a gravel drive in front of a huge palace. Attendants are helping us out, and we are about to go inside. My grandmother asks me to wait. She's fussing with my shawl and fixing my hair.

SK: Glance at your hand. Notice what you notice.

Georgia: I'm wearing a garnet ring.

SK: Is it the same exact ring you found recently?

Georgia: No, but the design is similar to the one I found in the antique store.

SK: How did you acquire the ring in your life in Hungary?

Georgia: I didn't. I'm borrowing it from my grandmother, and my mother is making a big deal out of it. Made sure I knew that this is the most valuable piece of jewelry our family owns. She wants me to wear it so I can make a good impression and seem like I have more to offer than I do. We go inside, and there's a ballroom, and a party's going on. They want me to make a good match to ensure our future.

SK: And do you?

Georgia: I feel overwhelmed. I don't want to be put on display, but I know our family is so poor, we need this to work. My mother is showing me the man she wants me to meet. He owns a nearby estate.

SK: Continue to explore these events and notice what happens. Do you meet him or not?

Georgia: I do. He seems to like me, actually, but there's another girl there who has a pushy mother, and he leaves with her.

SK: Fast-forward through your life to the next most significant event. Be there now. Notice if anything ever comes of it.

Georgia: I am in a bed, sick. I'm not going to make it.

SK: Did you ever marry?

Georgia: No. I'm sad [crying] for my mother and grandmother and worried about what they will do when I am gone, but I can't help being sick. It's not like I did it on purpose. I worry, though, about how they will get on without me. They are so very poor, and it's so cold, and the conditions there are substandard. I feel worse about leaving them than I fear dying.

SK: Float up and into the peaceful space between lives. Be there now. What lessons did you learn in your life in Hungary?

Georgia: To do your best for family.

SK: How does that apply to the life you're living now?

Georgia: We have a strong family structure. Family's everything.

SK: How has the garnet ring you found in the store helped you energetically?

Georgia: It reminded me of that connection and the bond we have that transcends time. The family wanted the best for me back then, and I'm lucky I have a great family now who also wants the best for me.

It's amazing to consider how and why our souls are attracted to different objects. We don't necessarily need to be connected to the exact items we once enjoyed to have Supretrovie bring us energetically back to our past.

Jerome Connected with His Aboriginal Past

Another amazing soul I met at an expo, Jerome, made a living as a percussionist. We began discussing the soul connection we all have to music in general, and he told me about a paranormal incident he experienced after receiving a didgeridoo for his birthday—an item that brought up a remembrance of ancient times.

"I'm a percussionist in a band, and way back in high school, my folks decided to surprise me with a didgeridoo. I always loved that thing, and actually I hadn't thought about this until you brought it up, but I do remember when I first picked it up and started to play it, I saw myself standing in the desert under the stars. It was super weird."

We did a regression to help Jerome access the source of his soul connection to music in general, and he went into a space where he uncovered the roots of his love for the didgeridoo:

SK: Where are you?

Jerome: The desert.

SK: Any idea of the date?

Jerome: I don't have that kind of linear thinking.

SK: Are you alone or with other people?

Jerome: I'm in a circle. It's night, and we have a fire going. Meat is cooking on spears. We're a brotherhood of men. Everyone has a task. We eat, and then we will share our toning with our voices and instruments. Every person has their individual spin on things—we all sound a little different, and each is contributing to the whole. We spend some time toning, then playing our instruments.

SK: Do you sense you work with a didgeridoo there?

Jerome: Not exactly like what I have now, but something similar, yes. It's a reed pipe that I hollowed out and let dry. It's much smaller than what I have in this life, but it sounds beautiful. I see this is why I love to play flutes as well as percussion.

SK: Do you do any percussion in that life?

Jerome: Oh yes, for sure. I've carved some of my own pieces and stretched hides over carved-out tree trunks. Awesome sound and resonance.

SK: How do you feel in this life?

Jerome: So present and conscious. I love it.

SK: How are you bringing that presence into your current life?

Jerome: It's not so easy in the modern world. I still love going off in nature on my own, and my life in Australia reminded me of that. I do my best to bring mindful awareness into my daily life. I think I'm a work in progress, though.

SK: How does your music relate to your experience as a soul?

Jerome: It's my purpose. I can help people through music. No words—just pure love. We need more love in our lives. That's how I do my part—that and helping build community through sound. It's so important to find ways to connect, and music is my way.

Jerome truly lived out his soul purpose in this life and others. I have not seen him since, but I am sure he's out entertaining people and building positive connections wherever he travels.

Nora Connected with the Ming Dynasty at a Museum in Shanghai

Family friend Nora, a deeply spiritual person, had a lovely home filled with gorgeous Asian art. She always talked fondly about her time overseas in her youth. I commented on her vast collection of art, including several vases that appeared to be hand-painted. To my surprise, she opened up about an uncanny experience that happened years earlier.

"My husband used to travel for work. He worked in the import business and took me to China and Japan several times when we were first married, before our children came along. I'll never forget visiting the art museums in Shanghai and seeing all the gorgeous calligraphy, vases, Buddhist figures, and artwork. I felt the connection to those areas ever since."

Nora had time on her hands and an open mind, so I asked her if she would like to undergo a past life regression to find out why she loved Asia so much. She said she started believing in reincarnation at a young age and agreed to try a regression to see what happened.

SK: Go back to the source event, to the original period when your soul first came to love Asian art. Be there now. Notice what's happening. What year is it?

Nora: 1440.

SK: Where are you?

Nora: China.

SK: Are you alone or with other people?

Nora: With others, lots of others.

SK: What are you doing?

Nora: Working, crafting, and making pottery. It's very strict. Everything must be done perfectly.

SK: How old are you?

Nora: Early twenties.

SK: As you experience the energy of the people around you, is there anyone you know from your current life?

Nora: I don't think so, but I can see that my whole family is there—my parents, siblings, and cousins. We all stay together.

SK: How has this experience affected your current life?

Nora: I've always been so attracted to Buddhist beliefs despite everything my parents taught me in my Christian upbringing. I also am quite the perfectionist. I can't stand to have my home or my life out of order. I strive for perfection. I don't always get things perfect, but I do try.

SK: Why did your soul return to China in your current life?

Nora: I believe I wanted the experience of connecting with my Buddhist beliefs, and thanks to my husband's work, I had that opportunity. I believe that happened for a reason, and I'm so grateful for that. I think more people should experience different cultures and belief systems so we can live without conflict.

Nora was surprised to learn she worked making the prized Ming pottery. I did some research into her dates, and sure enough, the Ming Dynasty ruled from 1368 to 1644 AD.[10]

The enduring connection Nora made with the Chinese culture, people, and art—triggered by her close proximity to museum artifacts from her earlier days—stuck with her for a lifetime and allowed her to enjoy a beautiful philosophical view of the world. She has since passed away, but her friendship remains a treasure I will continue to cherish.

Ivan's Coins Connect Him with Christ

Coin collector Ivan wrote me an email after reading one of my books. We wound up discussing a coin I encountered during my trip to the Holy Land called a widow's mite that people had during the time of Christ. The coins completely fascinated me. I found some for sale that were relatively inexpensive, but when I attempted to pick one out, it burned my hand. Not literally, of course, but the sensation jolted me so badly, I decided against bringing one home. Ivan mentioned that he owned several coins from the Holy Land and relayed his own bizarre experience:

"A while back, I acquired an ancient bronze coin associated with King Herod. The moment I touched it, I felt a surge of power shoot up my arm. It didn't hurt or anything like what happened to you, but the second I touched it, I had an image cross my mind of hundreds of people revolting in the streets. I had to put it down and go wash my hands. I pick up on all kinds of energy with the different coins I collect, but never anything as strong as that one. I've always loved coins, and I've been collecting some

---

10. History.com Editors, "Ming Dynasty," last modified January 10, 2018, https://www.history .com/topics/ancient-china/ming-dynasty.

really odd ones for years. Whenever I hold coins, I feel the energy of the past. I've always kind of believed that I must have seen them before in a past life and that they're meant for me to keep. For whatever reason, I want to be close to those memories. They give me strength."

The discussion resulted in Ivan's past life exploration into his connection with coins and specific moments in ancient times.

SK: Where are you and what year is this?

Ivan: Jerusalem in 40 AD.

SK: What's happening?

Ivan: I am an elderly man, scraggly clothes. I live in a shack.

SK: Are you alone or with other people?

Ivan: Other people are all around me, but I am not related to any of them. I think my family has passed. I sense I am a follower of Christ.

SK: Very good. Rewind and go back to the source event of your connection with Christ.

Ivan: It's 33 AD.

SK: What's happening in 33 AD?

Ivan: [Emotional] This is terrible. This shouldn't be happening. I want to stop it, but nobody can.

SK: Fast-forward again through those events and be back in 40 AD. How has your perception of what happened expanded since those terrible events?

Ivan: I have grown in my faith and know the truth when I hear it. I tried to connect with others who believe like I do, but many were put to death. None of this should have happened. I still try to share with anyone who will listen, but I am old now, and I know I won't live much longer. I can't seem to decide if being outspoken is better or if quietly discussing beliefs with people around me and remaining alive for a longer period of time to do so is better. I seem to want to live, though.

SK: Fast-forward to the very last day of your life in Jerusalem. Be there now. How is it that you pass away?

Ivan: Old age. I go to sleep. Nobody even notices I'm gone. I don't have any friends or family left. That's okay, though. I lived on my terms.

SK: Float into the peace between lives. How have these events influenced your soul journey?

Ivan: I am fascinated by the coins because they're one of the ways I connect to that time. I still consider myself to be very spiritual in my current experience. I follow my own beliefs and I am still devoted to Jesus.

SK: Were there other lives connected to the coins you've kept?

Ivan: Yes.

SK: Go now to the most important life you need to become aware of at this time. Be there now. What's happening and where are you?

Ivan: Rome. I'm a soldier. I hate my life. I had to kill people or be killed.

SK: What year is this?

Ivan: 29 BCE. I'm fighting a worthless battle. I'm stabbed and I die.

SK: How has this affected you in your current experience?

Ivan: I am a peaceful person. I do enjoy connecting with those times through my collections, though. I think they keep me grounded in the idea that wars are useless.

SK: Why did your soul choose to return after your life in Rome?

Ivan: I knew something important would happen, and I wanted to be a part of peace instead of war. I've lived through many wars, and I wanted something else.

SK: How do these experiences affect you currently?

Ivan: Knowledge is power. Understanding is critical to not making more mistakes, and I enjoy studying history so I can learn, and I do my best to avoid conflicts.

Ivan is certainly not alone in his emotional recollection of his past. I've run into many people who experience extremely poignant responses to and detailed memories of Christ's crucifixion. No doubt the experience is a critical part of their soul journey, and it strengthened Ivan's soul in the process.

Summing Up

Holographic impressions from long-gone memories can cling to objects. Have you ever experienced such a Supretrovie? In part 3 of the book, you'll have a chance to explore deeper connections to objects you may have used in the deep past.

Chapter Three

. . . .

GEM- & STONE-INDUCED SUPRETROVIE

MY NEWER READERS MAY not be aware of my deep connection to the gem and mineral kingdom. Growing up in Albuquerque, New Mexico; Phoenix, Arizona; and Colorado Springs, Colorado, our family always went out hiking, camping, and collecting rocks. My dad worked in the turquoise business and wound up managing the turquoise mines in Kingman and Bisbee, Arizona. Stones are simply in my blood!

Not until adulthood did I consciously recognize the profound healing energies inherent in all stones after a friend of mine, a Native American shaman, placed a piece of light green frosted Nevada fluorite on my forehead and told me to sit still because he wanted to show me something. Initially, nothing happened. The exercise seemed silly. Still, I waited patiently, and after a couple of minutes, healing vibrations bombarded me. I couldn't believe it!

The experience caused my curiosity to increase, so I began a personal project of placing other types of stones on my third eye to see how the feelings varied. Over time, the stones began speaking to me, telling me what they did and why. I ultimately created a wide collection of insights about what various gems and stones could do for body, mind, and spirit, which is the topic of many of my earlier books. I've come to understand that each stone is like a radio station. One might be like a jazz station, the other classical, and so on. Once you know what song a particular stone sings, you can tune in and allow that particular mineral to shift your frequencies to attract more of what you want in life.

A huge part of my business involves gem sales to the general public. I have a ton of fun watching people shop in the booths I've rented at various metaphysical fairs and expos over the years. Earlier in the book, I mentioned how fun it is to watch people look at my handmade art. Watching people gravitate toward gems and stones is just as fun and can also tell you a lot about someone, depending on which stone attracts them.

If I had a penny for each time I've seen people either fall in love with or be completely repulsed by a gem or mineral, I would have quite a fortune amassed by now. In addition to shifting unwanted influences to bring about healing, I've come to understand that gems cause spontaneous past life memories to emerge at least as often, if not more frequently, than other kinds of Supretrovie discussed in this book.

You would have thought that idea would have come to me right away, but it didn't. Not until years into my career of doing past life regressions did I finally come up with my current philosophy for the *real reason* people are so attracted to rocks. Yes, rocks are pretty and shiny, and we all love beautiful things, but external feelings and appearance are only part of the story. When someone is either repulsed by a stone or has an incredibly over-the-top reaction to it, they obviously need something the gem is offering in terms of healing. There's not always any easy way to know for certain what that is, but clearly the vibrations are affecting them in such a way that healing can occur. By shifting the frequencies within the energetic field, the stone raises the person's overall vibration and creates greater light and peace within them. At times, I've found that such over-the-top reactions can happen because the stone has awoken a deep memory of a past life in the same area where the stone is found in the world. The only way to confirm that is for the person to go on a past life regression to find out. This is yet another fascinating form of a geographical Supretrovie, only instead of flying somewhere on a vacation or business trip, the person has tuned in to the earth through the minerals found in that same place.

For example, all quartz crystals share the same fundamental geological properties of silicon dioxide. That's a given. Still, there's a huge difference in energy between a crystal from Arkansas and a crystal from the stunning island of Madagascar. Energetically speaking, the two are as different as night and day. Some of the truly special stones I've worked with over the years became known for their exceptional qualities, not because of *what they are*, but because of *where they are from* and the connection to the location and land where they're found. Another thing to consider is what the gem is called. Gemstones are often given trade names. Digging into the origins of minerals with unusual names will always reveal that the stone is simply named for a person who discovered it or for the place where it can be found. That research gives helpful clues as to why you're attracted to it. When people wear gems in jewelry or use them in healing, there's absolutely no doubt that at least half of the effects of any stone or mineral has to do with the origins.

I am so fortunate to have done all the traveling I've squeezed in during my current lifetime. Not everybody has that opportunity, and not everybody wants to travel. What I've found is that people don't need to venture out to tune in to prior incarnations. A gem or stone provides a strong personal connection to the world, a window into the past, and can often give folks a real blast from a past life that is every bit as profound as the experiences that happen to travelers. These next clients discovered that fact firsthand. Enjoy!

Ilona Returned to Atlantis

For years I've written about the stunning rare blue stone called Larimar, and I became the first person to bring the stone to Dallas back in the early 2000s to a very enthusiastic audience. Larimar is believed to have ties to the lost continent of Atlantis, and there's a theory that many people who live in the overly materialistic Dallas are reincarnated Atlanteans who are trying their best to overcome capitalism and get things right this time around. Some believe that Atlantis once thrived as a civilization until greedy villains destroyed everything. Whether or not that's true is obviously something we can't prove either way, but as a result—between that and my connections with the work of Edgar Cayce and his writings on Atlantis—I've attracted a lot of clients over the years who truly believe they were part of this once-great civilization and that the place is very much real. On the flip side, skeptics say Plato merely made up a fable for how humankind should strive to be and featured it in his book *Timaeus*.

I've had so many clients hold Larimar and burst into tears at my booths over the years, I can't even count them anymore. Larimar is a super high-frequency mineral named for Larissa, the daughter of the man who discovered it, and *mar*, which means "ocean." Anyone who goes on a Caribbean cruise will likely encounter Larimar, although sadly it gained such wide popularity that it's quickly becoming quite rare.

During her Caribbean cruise, like so many of my clients, Ilona became absolutely mesmerized by a stunning Larimar ring she saw in the gift shop aboard the ship. Something strange happened right after she bought it:

"I bought the ring in the jewelry store on the ship even though I told myself I was not going to buy anything, and definitely not anything that expensive. Oh well. You only go around once, right? Besides, I'd never heard of Larimar before. I had no idea what it even was. When the clerk handed it to me, I got lost inside the stone. I felt like I was in love, like my heart expanded all of a sudden. I had a feeling of total happiness beyond anything we can ever experience in real life. Not that I'm not happy, I am, but this went way beyond that. I became so emotional, I almost started to cry. I think you of all people will understand I'm not making this up.

After I put the ring on my finger, I had a vision of water all around me, and I felt peace like I'd never felt before. It was amazing. I felt like I'd been transported to another planet."

I understood exactly how Ilona felt and what she described. After first encountering Larimar at the Tucson Gem and Mineral show years ago, I dreamed of swimming with dolphins, and, just like Ilona and so many others, I felt a deep peace overcome my soul. Suffice to say, her story didn't sound strange to me at all, so we did a regression to uncover more.

SK: Where are you?

Ilona: This is definitely Atlantis, very early, during the good times.

SK: Are you a man or woman?

Ilona: A woman. I'm wearing a white, flowing gown, and I'm out on a land bridge on a remote island surrounded by beautiful water.

SK: How do you feel?

Ilona: [Crying] Happy.

SK: What do you do there? What's your purpose?

Ilona: [Pausing] I don't know. There is no such concept. We have very little conflict at this point, so we are simply being and experiencing oneness with all living creatures. We don't need healing because everything is in balance. We love. That's it.

SK: Very good. Imagine you can tune in to the same feelings you feel when you wear your Larimar ring. Fast-forward to the events connected with that feeling and be there now. Notice what's happening.

Ilona: I'm swimming. I'm free! I feel so incredible. There are dolphins, all kinds of tropical fish, coral, plants, and other wildlife. Everything is so bright and pure.

SK: Do you see the stone?

Ilona: No, not exactly, but I sense the energy is close to where I am. The stone has been on Earth for a long time, and it's near the area where I am now. The frequency is so high, it heals people just by being near it.

SK: Very good. Why did you choose to connect with this stone again in your current life?

Ilona: To remind me that we can achieve a better way of life for all people. We can rise above our current conflicts and learn to love again like we did in these early times. We have to trust and have faith and hang on to the feeling of unconditional love and peace.

SK: Nice. Anything else you learned? What lessons can you draw on from this early time as you move forward in your current life as Ilona?

Ilona: To love. Loving everyone and all beings is part of why we're here. Breaking through the illusion of separateness is our collective reason for being. We're all one. The sooner we understand that, the sooner we will have the peace we so desire.

SK: How are you using this information in your life and how does this early time relate to your soul purpose?

Ilona: I am here to hold the light and to show others how to love everyone they meet by doing so myself. I've had hard times in the past where I had to really work to remain calm, and this experience reminds me that peace is our birthright. Tranquility is the ultimate path to oneness and happiness for all.

I loved Ilona's message of hope and find this to be so timely, no matter where we are in life. The idea of loving each other is certainly meaningful. I haven't run into Ilona since our session, but I knew when we met that she had indeed tapped into a higher frequency, and I'm sure she'll use that to press forward on her personal mission of helping others through the challenges of life.

Hawaiian Sand Connected Hector to Current Life Bully

Hector and his wife went to the Big Island of Hawaii on a land tour to escape their hectic work schedules, and Hector became so enthralled by the black sand beach, he decided to bring some of the volcanic pebbles back to the hotel with him:

"Right before we arrived on the Big Island, the volcano overflowed onto some of the hiking trails, so the tour company postponed our walking tour until the following day. We decided to stay at the hotel and rest. Late in the afternoon, we heard another group had just returned from that area. I'm not necessarily the most patient person in the world, but I'm not reckless either. I would not have done anything that might have compromised our safety, but I told my wife I had to go over there, so we went. We arrived just before sunset, and once I got closer to the volcano, I felt really weird. Everything became quiet. I couldn't hear a sound, not even the dozens of people around us. I felt completely alone. I picked up a fistful of that volcanic sand, and I felt something in my hand. Like a burning feeling. Not like the volcano burned me, but more of an energizing feeling. I didn't think about the sand again until that night at the hotel. I had a dream I was in a large gathering dancing in a circle. I heard drumming and some kind of chanting. I woke up and felt so peaceful. I've always wondered why I felt so connected to that time and place. I've never experienced anything like it before or since."

Hector decided to find out whether or not he had a past life in Hawaii. Here's what happened:

SK: Travel back in time to the original moment your soul encountered the black sands of the area now known as Kilauea in Hawaii. Be there now and notice what's happening. What year is this?

Hector: 1538.

SK: Very good. What's happening?

Hector: I'm in a group gathered by a fire on the island. I see the volcano off in the distance. We're making offerings, chanting and praying.

SK: How do you feel?

Hector: Good. In tune with the land.

SK: Fast-forward to the next most significant event. Be there now. Notice what happens.

Hector: There's a battle. A neighboring group is attacking. I don't want to fight. I am not quick enough, and I am speared. I fall, and I'm dying.

SK: Go ahead and float into the peaceful space between lives. Be there now. What lessons did you learn in your life in Hawaii?

Hector: To be one with nature. Not to fight. There's no need.

SK: As you experience the energy of the people there, is there anyone you know from your current life?

Hector: [Thinking] Yes. I see a kid I went to school with in junior high. He's the one who stabbed me. He was the first bully I had as a kid.

SK: What lessons did the two of you learn in that life and in your current lifetime?

Hector: I wasn't mean to him, but I stood up to him in this life. I told him to go away, and he did. I learned that you can't just stand there and take abuse. You've got to stand up for yourself by saying something without hurting anybody.

SK: Why did your soul choose to return to Hawaii in your current life?

Hector: To connect with that land, the beauty. Reminds me of all the good things in the world.

No doubt, people are drawn to the places they loved in the past. Hector's soul learned from his past encounter with the bully, and he tapped into a peace he would carry with him throughout his life by visiting the true source event that explained his love for the stunning islands of Hawaii.

Kaia's Crystal Transported Her Back to Ancient Times

Recently, I've been offering some awesome crystals from Madagascar to clients online. The area is considered part of the lost continent of Lemuria, which is the subject of one of my earlier books. I love sending stones to people because it gives me the opportunity to send energy healing to them through the stones. I typically charge them up with healing light and symbology from some of the various healing techniques I teach.

After receiving her stone package in the mail, Kaia wrote to tell me about a peculiar experience she had with a crystal:

"The day the stones showed up, I had a super long day at work. I'm a restaurant manager, and we've been having to do deliveries around the clock and totally change how we do business because of the pandemic. I've been exhausted and stressed beyond belief. I pulled up in my driveway after dark, and as I did, I sensed something had changed. My house had a pulsing vibration around it, and I had a flash in my mind about the package. When I went out to check the mail, I found the package under some envelopes and flyers in the mailbox. I touched it and felt like a jolt of lightning burst up my arm. It should have scared me, but the feeling actually energized me. I took it inside and opened it up and there it was: that little Lemurian quartz you sent from Madagascar. It's such a sweet crystal! The other stones were neat, too, but that one took me by surprise. I held it and felt as though I had the weight of the world and all my burdens in life lifted off me by some unseen force. I've never had such a reaction to a stone or crystal before. That night, I slept with it, and I had a dream about floating deep inside a jungle, feeling happy and free. I've carried the crystal with me ever since."

I wrote back to Kaia, and we discussed her possible past life connections with the area, and she had a regression to find out more about her pleasant reactions to her new crystal:

SK: Where are you and what year is this?

Kaia: There's no time. I'm in a jungle area, the area I dreamed about. There are lush forests and exotic creatures everywhere. It's heaven on Earth.

SK: Other than these creatures, are you alone or with other people?

Kaia: I'm not sure. I don't have a sense of self like I do normally.

SK: Imagine there's a mirror floating down in front of you. Gaze into the mirror and notice what you look like.

Kaia: I'm nonphysical mist—a slightly purple-tinted light.

SK: What is your purpose for being there in this jungle?

Kaia: Myself and others like me are here to experience and learn about physical form, although we have not yet acquired that level of being. We want to be one with all things.

SK: Imagine you can fast-forward through this experience as a purple light. Notice what happens next. Do you stay in that same area or go elsewhere?

Kaia: We are moving around the world so quickly. I visit mountains, other forests, plants, and tiny microbial life-forms, connecting with all to understand consciousness.

SK: Move out of that experience as purple light and go into the space between lives. What lessons did you learn during your time as light?

Kaia: This is part of the soul evolution for myself and others around during these times. We will move forward and eventually into a physical form of our own. We could not feel any pain or any pleasant sensations during this experience, but we plan to move forward and do more.

SK: When you say "we," how many are you talking about?

Kaia: There's no way to quantify the numbers because we are one at this stage of development. We've not been separated at all.

SK: What lessons did you learn during your life as light?

Kaia: All consciousness is one. Separation is an illusion.

SK: How can you use that in your current life?

Kaia: For stress reduction, I need to remember this energy so I can bring that peace with me during my work hours. There is no need to worry or fear anything. We're all spirit, we're all formless. The body is an illusion, and we can become peaceful by remembering this source energy and being one with it.

SK: How will you do that?

Kaia: My crystal helps. Also, I can close my eyes and concentrate on the purple light and go back to that place. It's not hard to do. I must remember to keep connected in that way throughout my current life so I can be more helpful to others by remaining calm. When I relax and bring that calming energy to my work, I help other people find their own sense of peace.

Kaia's message of recognizing the connection to all things seemed to bring her a greater sense of peace. She wrote me after the session and said that by recalling what happened during her regression and keeping her crystal with her, she'd managed to drastically reduce her stress level. She said her coworkers seemed to react to her in a better way. Those whom she didn't get along with were more neutral to her, and dealing with various customers seemed to go smoother once she had her new realization about being one with all things. There's no doubt that when we change our inner vision, everything in our external world must change and shift in light of our new self-understanding. I know Kaia will continue to be a beacon of light for all who encounter her as she goes about her business.

Lenore Recalled Afghanistan After Holding Lapis

After writing several books about the father of holistic medicine, Edgar Cayce, I've had many clients who have been drawn to work with lapis lazuli. Sickly in youth, Cayce's family took him for hypnosis, and he fell into such a deep trance, he began relaying prophetic messages without recalling a word of what he said. Cayce gave people medical information and tuned in to their past lives. Cayce believed that everyone had karma they brought in from age-old experiences and that stones and gems could be used to alleviate past life challenges. Of all the stones in the over fourteen thousand readings Cayce did during his lifetime, he recommended lapis most of all. For that reason, I've worked with it extensively over the years and recommended that Lenore purchase a piece to alleviate her migraines. I didn't expect thirty-year-old Lenore to experience a Supretrovie in the Middle East from the lapis, which she wrote to tell me about a few days after purchasing the stone.

"I'm not sure if this lapis has anything to do with what I'm about to tell you or not, but while I was holding it, I went somewhere else—to a desert, and smoke swirled all around. It scared me, so I put the lapis down and haven't picked it up since. I'm not sure what that means."

We discussed the fact that she had perhaps picked up some impression about the stone's origins in Afghanistan, or that she might have been tuning in to one of her own past lives, so we set up a meeting to find answers.

SK: Imagine an energetic cord coming out of your solar plexus and connecting you with this lapis stone. Notice also that your spirit guide is taking out a big pair of golden scissors. When I count from three, your guide is going to cut the cord between you and this stone, releasing you from any unwanted energies. Ready? Three, two, one, and cut! Imagine a beautiful healing light is pouring down from above and moving through your stomach, into your heart, your arms and legs, and into your mind. Let me know when this feels better.

Lenore: Oh yes, this is much better.

SK: Very good. Ask your guide to tell you if the energy you picked up came from the stone itself: Yes or no?

Lenore: He's saying yes and no.

SK: Have him explain.

Lenore: I did sense some of that, but he's saying I have a connection to that area.

SK: Very good. Imagine you and your guide can go back to the true source event for your reaction to this stone. Be there now; notice what's happening.

Lenore: I'm there. In the desert.

SK: Are you a man or woman?

Lenore: A little girl. A few years old. A bomb is blasting our village. My parents are scrambling, trying to get us kids to shelter. It's terrible.

SK: What year is this? Say the first thing that comes to your mind.

Lenore: 1987.

SK: Surrounded by golden light, travel to the last day of your life in Afghanistan. Be there now. Notice how it is you pass into spirit.

Lenore: I'm killed by a blast. I don't know from where or how.

SK: Lift into the peaceful space between lives. Allow your guide to send a healing light down to all involved in this conflict. The light is getting brighter and brighter, lighter and lighter. Let me know when it feels better.

Lenore: [After a few minutes] Yes, it's better now.

SK: Ask your guide and your Higher Self if this situation contributes to the migraines you've been having. Yes or no?

Lenore: Oh yes. I am still carrying the stress around from this time. Also, my husband is in the army, and I remember my migraines happened a few years ago when they were talking about sending him over to Afghanistan. Luckily, they withdrew the troops, so he never went, but that's actually, now that I think about it, about the time the migraines started.

SK: Would you be willing to release that energy now that you know where it's coming from?

Lenore: Oh yes, definitely.

Lenore and I did more extensive healing and talking through releasing the residual residue of her former life in Afghanistan and the correlation to her migraines. She wrote to me a few weeks after our session and said she felt great improvement since uncovering her ties to her former life, and she had had a couple of milder episodes, but nothing like the severity she'd felt prior to the session.

We also talked about how the frequencies of stones can help resolve vibrational challenges in and around the body. When any stone is vibrating at one frequency and the body is at another, through continual connection, the body will eventually shift and get into a rapport and harmony with the stone, and various challenges have the potential of being relieved. I suggested that Lenore should continue to work with her lapis, even though that might seem difficult, until the frequencies between her body and the stone were in greater energetic alignment so she could become more peaceful, and hopefully her migraines could be eased. She agreed and said she could understand how that might be helpful. She said she kept the stone around always as not only a help energetically, but as a reminder of the family she lost and the life she once had in the Middle Eastern desert.

Ruby Connected Eli with His Life in India

Novice astrologer Eli hadn't been doing readings for very long when we met at a show. I had an intuitive sense he had talent, so I decided to allow him to prepare a forecast for me, which turned out to be well-done and pretty informative. During a break, he wandered over to my booth where, as usual, I sold different gems and stones, including some super awesome rubies from India. The moment he held one of my rubies, his demeanor completely shifted.

"Whoa! This is incredible! I have to have it! What is this?"

"Ruby," I said. "From India."

"I've always been drawn to India," he explained, pointing to the photo of Krishna he kept back at his table. "I'm certified in Western Astrology now, but the other method I've been curious about is Vedic."

I told Eli about my connections to Vedic astrology, my time as a transcendental meditation practitioner, and my two trips to India. "You probably had a life or two in India, which is why you're drawn to the energy of that ruby."

Eli decided to find out.

SK: Where are you?

Eli: India. I am seeing a map, and it seems like it's somewhere in the middle. I'm an astrologer. I study the various deities and do predicative readings for people in my village.

SK: What lessons are you learning in your life as an Indian astrologer?

Eli: We understand that all people and living beings are connected to the stars and everything we see in this exterior universe. There's no separation. We are intricately tied to the cosmos, and those connections can be recognized and predictions made to help people be happier.

SK: How does that life relate to your current incarnation?

Eli: I sense that it's taken me … I want to say a thousand years … to get back into doing this kind of work. I am happy I found astrology. I think it's an accurate way to use ancient knowledge to help others.

Once the session ended, I told Eli about some Vedic teachers I know, and he said he felt sure he needed to pursue the Vedic way of doing astrology in addition to using his current teachings. Interesting to note that Vedic astrologers prescribe gems and stones to clients to help vibrationally remedy weak planets in the astrological chart. The ruby helped awaken Eli's old memories and seemed to add inspiration for him to move forward and expand his abilities to help his clients.

Tess Survived a Crete Catastrophe
Brought On by a Necklace

After years of planning, Tess went on the trip of a lifetime to Athens and Crete, Greece, and wound up hospitalized and incapacitated for a month with a mystery illness. Could a past life problem be to blame?

"I saw your questionnaire, and I had to write in about something that happened to me years ago that, quite frankly, I've tried to forget. Several years ago, when I was in my thirties, I went with my then-husband on a Greek vacation. We flew to Athens initially and spent a night there, and everything was fine. The following morning, we flew over to Crete where we had a condo reserved for a week right on the ocean. Sounds like a dream, right? Wrong! Less than twenty-four hours after arriving, I came down with a high fever and started vomiting. My husband had no clue what to do for me. I hadn't even had a chance to get out much. My fever got so high, he had no choice but to take me into the emergency room, and they had to hospitalize me for several days. I don't remember much about any of that because I went unconscious, but once my fever subsided, I got well enough to at least go back to the condo. My husband decided it would be best to rearrange our flights and come home early, which we did, thank God, because the moment I got back to the States, I had a kind of relapse and wound up in the hospital again for almost a month. They quarantined me because nobody could figure out what I had, and again, I can't remember much about this because I was so out of it all the time. For some reason though, when I heard about your question about a past life, something made me wonder if that could have been part of the problem."

Physical illnesses are obviously quite real, but there's no doubt that sometimes those very real medical situations could be brought in from the holographic memory of things that happened long, long ago. I certainly found the idea intriguing. Tess decided to explore the matter further through a regression. Here's what happened:

SK: What year is this? Say the first thing that comes into your mind.

Tess: 678 AD.

SK: Very good. What's happening?

Tess: I'm there, in Crete. It's lovely. Absolutely gorgeous.

SK: Are you a man or woman?

Tess: A woman.

SK: As you experience the events in that life you had in Crete, is there anything that happened then that relates to the illness you experienced in your current lifetime? Yes or no.

Tess: Oh yes, definitely.

SK: Very good. Know you are still surrounded by a loving light. Go now into those events. Be there now. Notice what's happening.

Tess: [Gasps] Oh my God!

SK: What?

Tess: He's giving me a necklace and putting it around my neck. He gave me something just like that when we first arrived this time, and I forgot all about that. It's so similar!

SK: Is the necklace causing you a problem?

Tess: Yes and no.

SK: What do you mean?

Tess: I've been poisoned. My husband slipped something into my food or drink, but he may have rubbed my necklace in the stuff, too, just to make sure it did the job.

SK: Why did your husband poison you?

Tess: He thinks I cheated on him, but I didn't. He's paranoid.

SK: As you experience the energy of the husband you had in that life, is this anyone you know from your current lifetime?

Tess: Oh yes; it's my ex. The one who took me to Crete.

SK: What lessons did the two of you learn then that you've experienced again through your current lifetime?

Tess: He acted exactly the same way this lifetime. Even though I stayed devoted to him and loved him more than anything, he always acted afraid that I'd leave him and accused me of looking at other guys. He always thought I would break up with him. His paranoia ruined our relationship this time around. In Crete, it looks like he took matters into his own hands, even though he didn't have to do that.

SK: Float up and out of that body, out of that life. Be in the peaceful space between lives. As you gaze into your past, did you and this soul have other lives together that would explain his behavior?

Tess: Yes.

SK: Go to that moment in your soul's history when you were together another time and be there now. Where are you? What year is this?

Tess: This feels medieval. A mud hut, hard conditions. Early, like 1300s.

SK: What's happening?

Tess: He is my wife in that life, and I am a carousing husband. I am chasing anyone who moves and behaving badly. I see myself in one of those mead halls flirting with everybody.

SK: Float over those events and imagine you and your ex can speak to each other and explain what happened. Why have you had this dynamic?

Tess: His soul is apologizing for always being so paranoid. In our current life, he assumed I would do the same thing I did in the 1300s.

SK: Now that you understand his thinking, can you forgive him and release him?

Tess: Yes, absolutely, but I'll tell ya what. I think I still have that necklace sitting around somewhere, and I'm definitely getting rid of it as soon as possible!

Tess and I did a cord cutting with her ex, and although this all happened years before she and I met, the healing is still a powerful gesture for her own soul growth and will surely release unwanted energies and give her more peace and joy in her present incarnation. Our paths are often filled with opposing experiences so the soul can learn about different aspects of living, so when she accused him of irrational behavior, she had not ever considered that perhaps his feeling was not as ridiculous as she thought. He had simply been tuning in to a very old feeling from the past.

Summing Up

Gems and stones have been on our planet for millennia and will continue to be here when we are gone from this life and living our next. I hope this chapter gave you food for thought as you consider which stones you're attracted to and why. Who knows—you may have tapped into a past life! Stay tuned for part 3, where you will have a chance to find out!

Chapter Four

• • • •

SUPRETROVIE FROM CLOSE ENCOUNTERS

ONE OF THE MOST common kinds of Supretrovie happens when we find other people whom we've known in the past. During my initial research into the phenomenon of spontaneous past life memories, I didn't include this kind of experience, but I have since found it so common that I decided we must explore these familiar connections in order to have a well-rounded study of all the various ways we can connect with our soul history.

Back when I owned my travel agency, I had an incredible opportunity to go to Bali for a day as part of a longer Asian cruise. Bali has always held an allure about it, and I recall feeling a bit surprised that Bali was not as much like Hawaii as I'd expected. The people there are incredibly kind and welcoming, though, and I can certainly see why everyone loves going there. We walked through the gate at the Port of Benoa and went out to catch our bus to go visit a couple of temples. The traffic in Bali is hectic, and the homes, businesses, and personal temples, which are a required aspect of every single home on the island, were jam-packed together. Our driver sped down the road and screeched around curves, I assumed because we had only so much time to get to the opposite side of the island. At one point, I shut my eyes and cringed, praying to God that I would survive the journey.

I decided to open my eyes after our driver slowed for an intersection. I gazed out the left side of the bus at a neighborhood, and a swirl of energy washed over me out of nowhere. At the time, I couldn't tell whether I felt good vibes or trepidation, but the feeling stuck with me for several minutes. At first, I had no idea whether I had picked up on vibes in general or if the feeling had a more personal origin.

Bali is absolutely fascinating because the government requires every property owner to build a private temple at their home, so the city is stuffed full of monuments. Anybody could pick up on these vibrations to learn whether they had lived there in the past or not. That's probably why people fall head over heels in love with Bali. I've known several folks who actually uprooted their lives and moved there.

I soon discovered my soul connection to the area once our bus stopped. We toured two temples that day—Pura Taman Ayun, also known as the Royal Temple of Mengwi, and stunning Tanah Lot, a volcanic wonder right on the ocean. At the Royal Temple, I walked through the stunning grounds, and while moving up in the crowd to get closer to my tour guide so I could hear what he said, I became especially struck by his kind and pleasant demeanor, which is so common among everyone who lives there. I can't remember what we were even talking about, but I asked him a question and looked into his eyes. To my surprise and straight out of the blue, he smiled and said, "I've known you before."

Unlike the United States, many Bali residents are keenly aware of their past lives and believe in reincarnation. Most residents follow the Hindi religion. I gazed into his eyes and could definitely see what he meant. There was something so familiar there. "Yes, I see that," I told him.

Once I returned home, I went through an exploratory regression and saw myself in a mirror as an old Indonesian man. I lived near that same area I noticed on the bus, only in ancient times. My Higher Self showed me that same area, and the terrorizing bus ride flashed through my mind. Then the buildings faded away to the past life recollection of the area without any structures. I lived in a grass hut on a muddy swamp with my family. I noticed the rice paddies off in the distance and lovely details of my relatively peaceful existence. Surrounded by family, I saw my kids and grandkids. I realized the tour guide had been one of my little grandsons. In another brief vision, I saw myself teaching him how to fish.

Later in the book, you'll have a chance to do a mirror exercise yourself. It's quite interesting. Suffice to say, I don't have people tell me I've known them in past lives very often, but considering the palpable feeling of familiarity, combined with my pleasant regression and soul resonance for the loving people of Indonesia, I believe this sort of recognition is highly possible. As with everything described in this book, there's no way to know for sure, but the experience seemed validating enough for me.

Far beyond any mere occurrences of déjà vu, the clients in this section had visceral experiences when they encountered souls from the deep past whom they first met in times before their current incarnations.

Daphne Remembered Choking in the Philippines

The Philippines is a stunning island country known as a scuba diving paradise, which is exactly what Daphne decided to do with her friends when she had a blast from her past while eating fish in a local restaurant:

"I took a diving certification course with some friends from school, and we went off on an amazing adventure, living aboard a small boat and diving around the coral reefs for a week and a half. It was the best thing I've ever done in my life, and I loved the whole trip right up until just before we were ready to fly home. We rented a small boat and, I have to admit, a super cheap dive hotel in Manila, and we were wandering around the city eating street food. The second I locked eyes with the street vendor, I got a horrible feeling. I began choking really bad for no reason. I hadn't even taken a bite of my food yet, but I doubled over, and my friends had to slap my back to get me to stop. Eventually I felt better, and afterward I assumed I might have actually gotten some kind of foodborne illness from that fish, but I got on the plane, and once I came home, I felt totally fine. Nothing else happened. I wondered if I lived there in a past life, though."

Daphne's story certainly interested me, and she had a short regression to see if there was anything to her bizarre experience.

SK: Where are you and what year is this?

Daphne: I'm on an island in the Philippines. 1920s comes to mind.

SK: Very good. What do you look like?

Daphne: I can't tell, but I do sense I'm a woman.

SK: Are you alone or with other people?

Daphne: Seems like I am with a man. He's giving me a bad feeling. He's not a good man at all.

SK: You say he's no good. Is he mean to you personally?

Daphne: No, not at all. He treats me well, but I know he's in with some bad people. Into crime. I think he's killed people. You can see it in his eyes. He's made enemies.

SK: Fast-forward to the most significant event of this life that relates to your choking feeling you had on your trip to Manila. Be there now and notice what's happening.

Daphne: It's late at night and we are at our home. Some people break in and sneak into our room. Someone is strangling us. They won't shoot us because they don't want to make noise, but they're killing us.

SK: Why?

Daphne: Revenge comes to mind. My husband killed their brother is what I am hearing.

SK: Do you live through this?

Daphne: No.

SK: Float up and out of that body, out of that life, into the peaceful space between lives. Be there now. As you consider the energies of the people you knew in that life, is there anyone there you know in your current life?

Daphne: Yes, an old boyfriend. Nobody liked him. Everybody warned me about him, and I listened. I feel like people warned me about him in that life also, but that time, I did not listen. I am so glad I listened this time, because now I have a super fun boyfriend whom everybody likes, and I have a good life.

SK: Anyone else you know in your current life?

Daphne: This sounds nuts, but yes, it's him. The guy in the street market. I think he may have been the one who murdered us. He seemed familiar and may have been some criminal associated with my husband.

SK: What lessons did you learn in that experience in the Philippines?

Daphne: You can be a good person, but you become like the people you're with, and others will associate you with your friends, so it's important to choose wisely whom to spend your time and your life with.

SK: Why did you choose to go back there in this current life?

Daphne: I loved the area. Also, maybe so I could discover this about myself and heal from my past energy. I feel better about the whole situation now that I've figured this out. I won't wonder about it anymore.

Mob and gang activity remain common in the Philippines, so Daphne's account seemed plausible. Her soul apparently learned valuable lessons between that life and her current one, and although I haven't spoken to her since the session, I hope she remains well.

Dorian Met His Former Spouse at a Wedding

They say the eyes are the windows to the soul, so why shouldn't that be one of the ways we are transported instantaneously into our past life memories? That's exactly what happened when Dorian served as best man in his friend's wedding and glanced at one of the bridesmaids, who gave him a chilly feeling that he wanted to explore further.

"I'm only a few years out of college, and I like to date a lot, which everybody teases me about. My best friends are all married now, but I haven't met the right person yet. I recently went to another wedding, and when I saw Carla, I couldn't get over the strong feeling I had about her. Everybody thought she was so wonderful, but I didn't get it. Sure, she looked nice enough, but once I looked into her eyes, I didn't trust her from the get-go. My buddy kept reminding me Carla's single, and yeah, I found her attractive, but I still told him no. I could not go out with her, and I would not explore that as an option for even a second. Normally I'll give somebody a chance, especially someone who's so nice to me, but deep down something kept saying no. I'm curious why that happened. She's still single, from what I hear, and my now-married friends are having a party in a couple of weeks: a barbeque at their house. I know she's gonna be there. If there's something I could do now to make that easier for myself and understand what's going on with her, that would be awesome. Maybe I'm making it all up, maybe I'm nuts, but I don't want to be put in such an uncomfortable situation again. She told my buddy's wife she thinks I'm cute, so I have a bad feeling they're all still trying to set us up. I need answers."

Dorian definitely found answers to his questions about Carla in a time long ago:

SK: Where are you?

Dorian: In a pasture with mountains all around. Goats and sheep are grazing. I'm tending and feeding them. It's a peaceful life, but I'm worried something's going to eat them—wolves, maybe.

SK: Any idea what part of the world you're in?

Dorian: Up north, south of Russia. That place that begins with a U comes to mind.

SK: You mean Uzbekistan?

Dorian: Yeah, maybe. The area didn't have a name at that time because it was so unsettled and rugged.

SK: What year is this?

Dorian: 1402 comes to mind.

SK: Are you alone or with other people?

Dorian: I'm alone now, but I have a family around somewhere.

SK: Fast-forward to a moment when you're with the family. Notice what's happening.

Dorian: There she is! Carla's there. She's my wife! We live in a small cabin. She's there tending the fire.

SK: Very good. How do you feel with Carla in Uzbekistan?

Dorian: Good. She's cooking something over a fire. She weaves rugs and clothing from the skins I collect from my hunting. We keep lots of animal skins around for warmth—all we can collect. It's freezing up here and so primitive. We're all alone in the middle of nowhere.

SK: Is this a happy relationship or not?

Dorian: [After a moment] Uh, yeah. We get along very well. She's a sweet person and takes good care of me.

SK: Any children?

Dorian: No. Not yet. I sense she's younger than me and we have not been married very long.

SK: Fast-forward to the next most significant event of your life in the north and be there now. Notice what's happening.

Dorian: She's out picking berries and I'm in the cabin. I hear her scream, and I go running to find her. She's being attacked by one of those wolves. She's screaming. There's blood everywhere. She's trying to save our sheep. The wolves got one of them and they're dragging it off, but I shout and scare them away, so the one attacking her lets go and they all leave.

SK: What happens next?

Dorian: I carry her into the house and try to stop the bleeding, but she doesn't make it.

SK: Fast-forward to the very last day of your life in the north and be there now. How do you pass into spirit?

Dorian: I live a fairly long time after that. I'm alone. Very depressing. I eventually become ill and pass away.

SK: Move into the peaceful space between lives. What lessons did you learn in your time in the north?

Dorian: You can't count on anyone. You come into this life alone and you leave alone.

SK: How does that affect you now?

Dorian: This may be why I'm the last of my buddies to settle down. I have a deep-rooted fear that things won't go well if I do.

SK: Do you want to change that or not?

Dorian: I think so, yes.

SK: Was this the only time you knew the soul whom you call Carla?

Dorian: No.

SK: Go back to another life when the two of you were together. Be there now. Notice what's happening.

Dorian: She's my wife again. We have some kids and are very happy together, just like we were before.

SK: What year is this?

Dorian: 1200s. We're in the desert this time.

SK: Fast-forward through that life. How do things go for the two of you?

Dorian: The life itself was tough compared to how we all live now. No modern conveniences, harsh weather, always fighting to survive and making sure we had enough food and fresh water. We had some animals again. This time I passed away first. She stayed by my side when I died.

SK: What lessons did the two of you learn then?

Dorian: Family. The importance of family.

Once we finished the session, Dorian seemed a bit confused. He expected to confirm that Carla was a monster whom he should avoid because she had somehow harmed him in the past, when in fact nothing could be further from the truth. He loved Carla on more than one occasion. The fear of losing her had prevented him from even taking her out for a coffee. After gathering his senses and wrapping his mind around this new paradigm, he expressed the fact that he may now be open to getting to know her better.

Like all of us, Dorian is free to make his own choices. Not everybody wants a relationship. Once he went through the regression and so clearly saw his feelings for Carla firsthand, Dorian seemed to have a profound sense of missing out on something significant by staying single. After he mentioned that he may want to change that feeling within himself, we did a healing to release the old fears of his past so he could move forward. Dorian left the session with a greater sense of peace about relationships in general and a newly opened mind in relation to Carla herself.

I asked him to keep in touch and let me know how it went at the party. He sent an email to let me know he spoke to Carla extensively and they planned to go to dinner soon. I haven't heard from him since, so I hope the date and both of their futures went well.

A Past Life Nuisance Became Helene's Horrible Boss

People spend a shocking amount of their lives working, and like so many of my clients, Helene came to see me thanks to trouble at her job. Her new supervisor caused her unnecessary stress and trouble, even though she claimed she did nothing to provoke him.

"The moment I looked at the guy, I had a bad feeling. He seemed like trouble. Why, I couldn't tell you. I've tried everything I can think of to get along, but for reasons I can't explain, it seems he has it out for me. I don't have enough time to tell you all the little things he's done to get under my skin, and I know I should be a better person. Believe me, I'm trying. Suffice to say, he's been a total nightmare. We work in one of those big call centers. The biggest problem is the fact that he never gives me good ratings on any of my calls, even though I've been in this department longer than any of my coworkers. My reviews affect my pay increases, which I've received regularly each and every year I've worked here. If I can't get to the bottom of this, I'll have to quit, which I hate to do because I like my job, but I can't take much more of this situation. If he won't stop, he'll ruin my reputation and my chances of getting a better job elsewhere in the future. That's not what I want, though. I don't want to leave the company. I have seniority and a lot of good friends there. I need help!"

Helene found that the trouble with her new supervisor originated in the past:

SK: Where are you?

Helene: Vienna, Austria.

SK: What year is this and what's happening?

Helene: It's early 1700s. I'm a very wealthy woman, and right now, I'm walking through the city.

SK: Is there anyone you know from your current life?

Helene: Oh yes. He's there. I see him. He's a dirty old creep walking through the streets talking to himself. He lives on the street. I think he's homeless.

SK: Could you help him or not?

Helene: I'm afraid of him. He's too unstable. I wouldn't even know where to begin to help him, so I try to go the other way and get away from him.

SK: Fast-forward through these events and notice what's happening.

Helene: I made it to my carriage, and I return to my estate and tell my husband all about what happened. He's telling me that the man is the older brother of someone we know.

SK: How does that change how you view him?

Helene: I do feel bad. We're talking about the cold and how the snow will be coming soon. He had a head injury of some kind not too long ago, and if we don't help him, he won't make it through the winter. My husband sends some of our staff to collect him. We fix him a place on our property where it's warm and he will be safe and fed.

SK: How does it make you feel knowing you saved him?

Helene: Better. We had a doctor give him something to calm his nerves, and he is actually recovering to some degree.

SK: Is this the first time you've known him?

Helene: No. I also knew him in the Middle East. I want to say 1300s. I live in an old city. Seems like it's somewhere in Iraq. There he is again, raggedy and dirty. I am wealthy, clean, composed, tailored, organized. I am an older woman in that life, refined and soft-spoken. I don't go out without my husband, so he doesn't bother me then.

SK: Fast-forward to see what happens.

Helene: He crosses my path again, and I see people treating him cruelly. I ask my husband to persuade the people to leave him alone. He speaks to them, and they do, because we are respected.

SK: Does he thank you and your husband for that?

Helene: No. He doesn't have the capacity to understand. We get him some food and try to help him.

SK: Does it work?

Helene: No. We found him a safe place to stay, but he wouldn't be still. He escaped, and someone found him dead not too long after that. One of the cruel people bothering him killed him despite what my husband and I tried to do. They didn't understand him. Some thought he was cursed, and they believed they had to get rid of him.

SK: Any other times you knew him?

Helene: Oh yes.

SK: What year is that and what happened?

Helene: BCE comes to mind. 600?

SK: Where are you in 600 BCE?

Helene: A grassy plain in the middle of nowhere. I'm a young girl. He is there again. A wanderer. My father feeds him and he moves on.

SK: Move up and out of that body and into the peaceful space between lives. What lessons did you learn with this other soul that you are currently reliving in this current time?

Helene: To help people no matter what their circumstance. In my current life, he is the wealthy one, and I am not poor of course, but I am not at his level. He wants to look down his nose at everyone, but that's wrong. I hope he can learn.

I found the challenge between Helene and her boss to be troubling because one would assume you would like someone who tried to help you through the ages. We did a healing between Helene and her boss's Higher Self where she talked directly to his Higher Self to find more answers about the reason he treated her so poorly.

SK: What is he telling you?

Helene: He is angry and doesn't want charity. He said I dishonored him by giving him handouts. In this life, he's amassed a fortune on his own, supposedly after coming from humble beginnings. When he sees me, he remembers these other lives, and he wants nothing to do with that old energy. He is wealthy now, and that's it.

SK: What resources could you give him now to make him feel at least more neutral toward you?

Helene: Respect, autonomy, self-reliance, and peace.

SK: Very good. Imagine you and your spirit guide can give all those things to him now, and allow a healing light to move through him. Let me know when you both feel better.

Helene: [After a moment] Yes. Better.

SK: Imagine you can both notice an energetic cord that represents all things in the past connecting you. In a moment, your spirit guide will cut that cord so you can begin anew with none of the energy from those former times. Ready? Your guide is cutting that cord now.

Helene: That feels better.

I wanted Helene to let me know how things went because I had high hopes that her situation would improve. Sure enough, the tension lessened, and she wrote a second time to let me know he had actually recommended her for a job promotion into another department where they would not be around each other as much. That would probably be a good thing in the end, and also, he energetically released his resentments, and the two parted on good terms.

I can't stress enough how empowering it is to send healing to others in this way. Releasing people from transgressions from former lives and blessing their path into the future can make huge positive shifts for everyone involved.

Cole's Fear of Water Had Ties to a Past Life Teacher

Nothing works better on phobias than past life regression. I can't count the number of times a quick trip into the past remedies deep-rooted and unexplained fears and banishes them forever. Cole wanted to explore why he hated water and spent his childhood avoiding pools and water in general at all costs:

"This isn't life-threatening or an emergency or anything, but I have missed out on some fun events in the past because I won't go near the water. I wouldn't have cared and probably wouldn't have even wanted to look into this at all, except that my wife and I had a chance to go on a beach trip with a bunch of couples last summer, and I said no. I felt bad for having to disappoint her, so I want to see if I can get this resolved."

Cole's desire for self-improvement impressed me. As expected, his trip to the past brought up a memory of a familiar friend he hadn't thought about since childhood:

SK: Where are you?

Cole: A ship.

SK: What year is this?

Cole: 1509.

SK: Where are you?

Cole: I'm not sure. I'm from somewhere in Europe. England maybe, but we're not there now. We're in the middle of the ocean.

SK: Is this the source event of why you avoid water?

Cole: Yes.

SK: Fast-forward through these events during your life on a ship in the 1500s. Remember, you are surrounded by a golden protective light. Notice now what happens to cause your fear of water.

Cole: We passed near some islands and thought we were in the clear, but our ship hit a rock, and now there's a hole in the hull. The captain is shouting to everybody to let us know what happened. We're all running down into the belly and chipping in to bail the water out, but we can't do it fast enough, and we're going down. There's nobody to help us.

SK: Anyone there who feels like someone you know in your current life?

Cole: Whoa! There's my science teacher from junior high. He was a cool old dude, a real intelligent man I admired. I remember the first time we met. He always liked me and encouraged me back then, which is one of the reasons I became an engineer. He had a real influence on my life. I doubt if he's even alive anymore. He's the captain of the ship. He's coming around and trying to calm everyone; he's apologizing, too, but it's not his fault. There's nothing he could've done about that rocky patch. He couldn't have stopped it.

SK: Imagine you can float through the last day of your life and into the peaceful space between lives. Be there now. What lessons did you learn in that life on the ship?

Cole: Teamwork.

SK: How has this situation affected your ability to be in and around water?

Cole: I just don't do it.

SK: Is this the only event that's preventing you from going in and around water? Yes or no.

Cole: Yes.

We did a clearing on the situation, bathing all involved in the shipwreck in healing light, and then Cole went into his future, where he saw himself floating in a swimming pool. A few weeks after our session, he emailed to say that he did what he said he would and tried out his neighbor's pool. He said he felt good, and although he didn't stay in the water for long, Cole made a huge step forward compared to where he had been only a short time earlier. Changing perspective and agreeing at a soul level to release the past can make a huge difference in life, as Cole found out.

Sondra Recalled Her Banker from the Icy North

Sondra had a fairly conservative demeanor for someone interested in past lives, so I was especially curious to see why she sought a regression. In her mid-eighties, she told me about an encounter she'd had recently with a man who worked at her bank:

"I'm happily married," she explained rather defensively. "I'm ashamed to share this story, but I had to go to my bank a couple of months ago to make an inquiry about my account. I waited for someone to come out, and the young girl took me back to see the branch manager, whom I'd never met before. I began speaking to this young man, who is probably younger than my own grandson, and when I looked into his eyes, I felt like I'd known him forever. Now, whenever I go into the bank, he's always in the lobby, almost like he knows when I'll be there. We talk about all sorts of things. He's become a good friend despite our age difference. I mentioned this to one of my closest friends, and she suggested I get in touch with you to see if we may have known each other before in another lifetime."

Sondra displayed the same characteristics of a teenager in love for the first time and clearly didn't appear comfortable with her feelings at all. She had a tough time admitting any of this to me, and I did my best to reassure her. Sondra's hunch proved correct. Here's what happened:

SK: Where are you and what year is it?

Sondra: 1400s. I'm on a vast piece of land living in a tiny cabin. It's up north, very cold. Norway, maybe.

SK: Are you a man or woman?

Sondra: A woman.

SK: Are you alone or with other people?

Sondra: I'm with my husband and three small children.

SK: As you experience the energy of your family, are there any of them who feel familiar to you?

Sondra: Oh yes. My banker. He's my husband.

SK: How do you feel in that life with him?

Sondra: Happy. Content. A simple life.

SK: Is this the only time you've known each other?

Sondra: No.

SK: How many other times have you known him?

Sondra: Three.

SK: What relationship did you have with him in the other three lifetimes?

Sondra: We were married and always happy.

SK: Is it important for you to visit any other times? Yes or no.

Sondra: No, not necessarily.

SK: Float over the last day of your life in Norway in the 1400s. Be there now. How do you pass into spirit?

Sondra: I'm very old by the standards of that time. My husband died long ago. I'm lonely except for my children.

SK: Leave that body and float into the peaceful space between lives. Be there now. What lessons did you learn with this soul you know as a banker in your current life?

Sondra: Respect and love. Caring and simplicity.

SK: Why did you choose to meet up again in this life?

Sondra: Our timelines are not right in this period. We will see each other again one day. We stopped to say hello is all. The soul is endless. We meet friends along the way, and it's all good.

Sondra's story fascinated me and reminded me of *The Curious Case of Benjamin Button* with Brad Pitt. It's a film about a man who gets younger over time and misses out on his one true love as she ages and passes on. We've likely had many soul mates over many lifetimes, and we encounter each in new ways as we make our way through our life journey.

Basil Found Business Success with His Cherished Nephew

After a tough breakup, Basil relocated back to his hometown and decided to have a past life regression to help him decide what to do next. Before we began, we discussed some of the important people in his life, and he mentioned he had a tight bond with his nephew, partly because he had a hand in raising him.

"My younger sister got pregnant in her teens and by then my dad had already passed away. When my nephew was born, I was right there with him and became like a father figure to him. I never had kids of my own, so he's like my son. One of my ideas is to help him start a business he's been asking me about, but I want to make sure I'm doing the right thing by him. I want him to succeed, so I hope I can find answers to help me decide if this is what I need to do or whether I should steer him in the direction of getting a job. I would do anything for him, but it's me I worry about. I don't think of myself as a businessperson, and I want him to have a better life than I had, so any information on that would be great."

SK: What year is this and where are you?

Basil: 1863 somewhere in the Midwest. I live on a farm with my family.

SK: Anyone there feel like someone you know in your current life?

Basil: My sister's there. She's one of my daughters, and my nephew is my son. I have three kids total, but I don't know the other child or my wife.

SK: Fast-forward through important events in your life on the farm. What happens?

Basil: I teach my son everything I can—hunting, fishing, how to tend the crops. He's my sidekick. I don't see my girl around, and I am thinking that the other child must also be a girl because it seems like they're with my wife, so I spend all my time with my son.

SK: Go to the next most significant event in your life on the farm. Notice what happens.

Basil: I'm in town trying to sell my crops. People try to rip me off. My son is older, and he's stepping in to negotiate. He's better at it than I am.

SK: How does that apply to your current life?

Basil: He's still sharp as a whip. I should put him in charge of the business side while I stay on the production side. We're still a great team.

SK: Is this the only life where you two knew each other?

Basil: No.

SK: Imagine you can visit another life with you and your nephew that would further give you insights into what to do about your business. Be there now. Where are you?

Basil: The woods. I want to say Ireland.

SK: What's happening?

Basil: I'm outside my cabin. I have a small business there, but it's burning to the ground. I lose everything.

SK: Is your nephew there?

Basil: He's my son again. I manage to get my family out safe, but I left a fire on, and it's my fault they almost died, and now we're homeless and have nothing.

SK: How does this relate to what you're doing in your current life?

Basil: That fear's still there that I will mess this up and ruin everything. I can't let that happen.

We did some work to help Basil forgive himself and realize that everyone makes mistakes, and we discussed the other life where he clearly had an amazing partnership with his then-son by recognizing each person's strengths and weaknesses. The epiphany on whether to proceed came when he traveled into his current life's future to see the business:

SK: Where are you?

Basil: In our shop. It's a fish and tackle store, a homegrown hunting resources place.

SK: What's happening?

Basil: Steven's there—my nephew. He's in the back working on orders and doing the books, and I'm in the shop part with a customer, answering questions about fishing lures.

SK: How do you feel?

Basil: Awesome. This kid has such a great head for business, and I really enjoy our customers. It's the best thing I've ever done.

SK: What does Steven tell you about how grateful he is that you decided to do this with him?

Basil: He does tell me that a lot, and I try to get him to stop. He's a good kid, and he will do great at whatever he does in life.

Last I heard from Basil, he and his nephew were looking for space to rent. He tapped into his past life gifts and realized that everyone has their own talents. By joining forces with his nephew, the two of them seemed to be headed into a promising future.

A Forever Friend Became Talia's New Coworker

Talia worked as an office manager at a busy law firm. Her employer valued her tenure, and she often had to help train new associates joining the firm. In her spare time, she enjoyed quilting and knitting and had recently experienced something startling.

"My boss called me out of my office and asked me to join him and one of our new hires so I could help her get situated, and when I went to meet her, I shook her hand, looked in her eyes, and almost passed out. I saw a movie play in my mind about sewing. I don't know what's going on, and of course I didn't tell her about it because I didn't want her to think I'm insane. I took her around that first day and kept having a feeling that I know this woman. Like we were very old friends. I tried running through my whole life, trying to figure out if I knew her in elementary school or junior high or something, but I can't figure it out. One of my friends suggested we may know each other from a past life. I never thought of that before. Since then, we've gone to lunch a couple of times, but I still don't know her well enough to tell her I believe in all this stuff. I may someday, but for now, I have to keep it to myself."

Talia soon discovered her insights were more on the mark than she could ever have imagined:

SK: Where are you?

Talia: Lithuania?

SK: Very nice. What year is this?

Talia: 1820.

SK: What's happening there in Lithuania?

Talia: I'm standing next to a rock in the woods. I'm picking up pebbles with another lady who's wearing thick, heavy brown shoes. She's a good friend. We're relaxed and carefree.

SK: Is this woman anyone you know from your current lifetime?

Talia: Oh yes—it's Jenny, our new associate. She's still just as caring now as she was back then.

SK: Fast-forward to the next most significant event in that life. Be there now. Notice what's happening.

Talia: We're in a room sitting by a fire and stitching up clothing. Our children are running around playing, and we're talking, happy.

SK: Is this the first time you two were together?

Talia: No.

SK: Go back to an earlier time when you were together. Be there now. Notice what's happening.

Talia: I'm in a wood cabin with a warm fire. It feels like 1740s. I'm cooking for my husband. He's a kind man, very simple. He's in work clothes. I'm baking bread. It feels close to where we lived in the other life. Poland, maybe? I'm not sure. I don't think it had a name back then. Oh, and Jenny's there. She's our baby daughter.

SK: How old is she?

Talia: [Thinking] Almost two.

SK: What lessons did the two of you learn in that life?

Talia: We had a very good time. I love my husband; he's kind, and we have a relatively comfortable life. I learned that relationships are important. Love is important. Peacefulness and love are the most important things anyone can experience.

SK: Very nice. Any other lives with the two of you?

Talia: Yes.

SK: Be there now. Where are you?

Talia: So early. This feels like another small farm. I'm in a cabin again. [Gasps]

SK: What's happening?

Talia: This is the place! This is the place I saw in my head when Jenny and I first met.

SK: Very good. Where are you?

Talia: Scotland comes to mind. This is earlier, like 1580.

SK: What is so significant about your life in Scotland?

Talia: I'm a very old woman. There's a child there; she may be my grand-daughter. We're all gathered around knitting and looking at pieces we created. It's peaceful again.

SK: Why do you create all these things?

Talia: We raise sheep, and it's so cold there, we have to learn to use all our resources. The knitting and sewing are part of our culture and community. It's just what we do. We use the resources we have available, and it's how our community stays connected. Friendships are built that way.

SK: What lessons are you and Jenny learning together in many lifetimes?

Talia: Loyalty, love, and friendship.

SK: Will you tell her about this regression?

Talia: No, not right away.

SK: Why did the two of you get together in this current life?

Talia: To connect more as friends rather than as caregivers. I don't know enough about her yet to know if she would be open to these ideas, but for me, it's nice to know I have a real friend in her. I know no matter what, she's someone I can trust.

Doctor Saved Angus in a Bloody Past

Like so many on the path, Angus became increasingly interested in spirituality after a near brush with death. He sought a past life regression to deepen his understanding of why he survived and what his purpose is for the remainder of his current lifetime. His accident had been such a close call, anyone in the same situation would have undoubtedly been on a soul searching journey. Not only did Angus describe an otherworldly trip to the space between lives, but a keen sense of familiarity he felt for the doctor who saved his life:

"Five years ago, I got in a head-on collision when a drunk driver swerved over several lanes of traffic and hit my pickup. I never saw it coming, and I'm lucky to even be here. I broke my collarbone, crushed my femur, and collapsed one of my lungs in the wreck. They pronounced me dead at the scene, and I came back after going into the light and being told it wasn't my time. I spent several days in the hospital in a drug-induced coma. Aside from all that, my doctor was the first person I saw when I came to. He was a fairly young guy, probably in his mid-thirties. I will never forget the first time I saw him. I looked into his eyes, and my mind started flashing back to wars and famines. I thought it might be the drugs at first, but after all I've been through, and now with everything I've experienced after having my near-death experience, I believe there was more to it than that. I never told the doc, of course, because I didn't want him to think I had an irreversible head injury or whatever, but I knew that guy before. I've seen him a couple of times for follow-up appointments since they released me from the hospital, and I've always wondered where we were together in the past."

Anyone who goes through such a traumatic event as Angus would certainly feel an overwhelming sense of gratitude and connection with the people who worked so hard to save them. Could that connection also be tied to a far older event? Angus and I did a regression to find out. Here's what happened.

SK: Where are you and what year is this?

Angus: Massachusetts, 1775.

SK: What's happening?

Angus: I'm a soldier in the Revolution.

SK: Very good. Surrounded by golden light, allow yourself to move through these events. Notice what's happening.

Angus: I'm hit. I fell by a tree. Someone is coming to help. It's one of my fellow soldiers. That's him. The doctor. I'm not sure why he even bothered. I hear people all around telling him to leave me, but he won't. He carried me on his back to a makeshift hospital and worked on me.

SK: What happens next?

Angus: He stitched me up, and I might have actually pulled through, but I've got a fever, and I pass on a few days later.

SK: Go ahead and do that now. Float into the peaceful space between lives. Be there now. Is this the only time when your soul knew the doctor?

Angus: No.

SK: Return to the source event when you first met the soul whom you know as your doctor. Be there now. What year is this?

Angus: I want to say the 800s.

SK: Very good. Where are you?

Angus: It's cold. I'm on a wooden boat with cloth sails, rowing. Everybody's covered in furs. Snow's blowing all around. It's brutal outside.

SK: Fast-forward and arrive at your destination. Where are you?

Angus: We landed on a shore. We're unpacking our gear. A man is passing out dried fruit and fish, and we're fueling up so we can get going.

SK: Where are you headed exactly?

Angus: I'm not sure. South of there, somewhere, we heard there are resources we want. We're planning to conquer whomever we find.

SK: How many people are with you on the boat?

Angus: A dozen or so.

SK: Anyone feel familiar to you?

Angus: Yes, the doc's there, too. He's one of the men.

SK: What is your rank within this group?

Angus: Both of us are just workers. We're following orders. We don't have a choice to be doing this, because if we didn't go to battle, we would have been punished. Our land is barren, so if we don't make these moves, we're afraid we'll die out, so it's not only greed, but survival that's motivating us.

SK: Fast-forward through the events. Notice what happens.

Angus: We eat and gear up and head south. We're not expecting to meet much opposition, and we're in for a huge surprise. There's a brutal group who is fighting back and fighting hard. A good half of our men are down. Doc's one of them. I'm nearby, and I drag him to safety.

SK: What happens next?

Angus: It's night, and we're in camp. I'm tending to him and have him lying near the fire. He may pull through.

SK: Fast-forward and see what happens.

Angus: He actually makes it, but he's not the same. Really weakened. Our mission fails, and we retreat and return to the north with what little we managed to steal. Back in the village, people are glad to see us, but we don't have much to offer. Some metals and pottery, but we needed food, so it's not enough. Some of the others brought more from their trips to the south, but still, we're going to have to keep going and moving out in order to live.

SK: Fast-forward to the last day of this life in 800. Be there now and notice how you pass into spirit.

Angus: I'm speared in the gut out on a battlefield again. My friend is by my side, trying to help, but I'm much older than him, and I don't make it.

SK: Float out of that body, out of that life, into the peaceful space between lives. What lessons did you learn in those early times?

Angus: Survival requires sacrifice.

SK: And what lessons were you and your friend learning as souls together?

Angus: I think we were brothers. We learned to have each other's backs no matter what.

SK: Is this life and your life in the 1700s the only two lives you have had together?

Angus: Oh no. We've had several. We're usually brothers, and we come together to take care of each other.

SK: Why did your soul choose him as your doctor in this life?

Angus: I don't know if another doctor would have saved me or not. Maybe. He came in this lifetime just for that purpose. He wanted to make sure I lived.

SK: Do you think you will become friends down the road?

Angus: Even if I never see him again, which I probably won't since I haven't run into him since my last appointment a few years back, he is someone I trust with my life. If I do wind up coming back in another future life, I hope to see him again, or at least people like him who really care about me. You don't have many people in your life like that. I'm lucky he showed up when he did.

Angus continued with his spiritual pursuits. Last I heard from him, he kept busy by going out and sharing his experience from his accident with others through talks. He went on an incredible journey of healing and self-transformation that we can all learn from.

Summing Up

The longer I live, the more I believe we come to each life experience with a plan of whom we will meet and what we will do. Not every second is preordained, mind you, but we definitely choose the souls we want to meet to help us grow and learn to become better people, or those we loved come to act as part of the wider support system every person needs during the life journey. I hope this section gave you cause to recall some of the people you've encountered in the past whom you immediately recognized on a soul level.

PART TWO

· · · · · · · · ·

GUIDED JOURNEYS

NOW IT'S YOUR TURN to explore your own instances of Supretrovie in various areas, be they geographically induced from places you've been or triggered by objects or the deeper connections to people you've met.

One of the most valuable aspects of journey work and regression in general is the fact that often you get incredibly surprised by what you uncover during these processes.

I've written out several exercises in this section that you can use. I highly recommend trying one of the many recording apps you can get for your phone. Record the scripts, read them back to yourself, and enjoy the revelations you'll discover.

Chapter Five

• • • •

MEMORY JOGGING, TUNING IN & PSYCHOMETRY

TO GET YOU READY to explore your past life connections to various people, places, and things, we will do several helpful healing and memory jogging exercises, and you will learn how to do psychometry—gleaning intuitive insights from objects. You probably haven't stopped to think about the fact that you are connected energetically to the items you keep. In fact, you may find it silly to think you may have past life connections to your stuff. That's fine! Believe me, I would never have considered this either until I began digging into this information. We are attracted to the people, places, and, yes, the things we have known before. That's what I believe, and that's what I've found to be true for many of my clients. This section will help you explore this phenomenon and get to know yourself better than ever before.

One important point I must emphasize as we move into our work on memory and psychic sensing is this: don't think too much. If you're like me, you may enjoy overanalyzing every little thing. When practicing intuitive exercises, it's always best to be totally open and allow pictures, thoughts, and feelings to bubble up from some space outside of yourself while trying not to judge. Easier said than done, I know, but keep this important tip in mind as we delve into the following exercises that are designed to get you in touch with the origins of items you may have encountered in past lives.

We will begin with the memory jogging processes. Each time I worked with clients regarding Supretrovie, I noticed that for the most part, they all shared a common trait—the memories were hard to recall. Many responded to a survey I sent out and mentioned that it took them a few days to recall what happened so they could even respond to my survey, even though at the time, they felt the incidents were meaningful in their lives. The memories are hard to recall because for most people, the things that happen to them seem so out of the norm, many assume they are some figment of their overactive imaginations. In reality, that's not the case at all. These flashes are giving people real insights into who they really are and who they have been throughout the ages.

In the first part of this chapter, we will begin the journey to assist you with uncovering your own past life memories by helping you recall any weird thoughts and feelings that occurred to you at some moment in the past. Once that's done, we will move forward to the regression section in the next chapter, and by then, you will have a clear vision of which memories you want to work on. Let's get started!

Journal to Bring Up Deeply Embedded Memories

I've been journaling personally since childhood. There's nothing more beneficial to your soul than sitting still for a few moments and capturing your thoughts on paper. To get to the deepest aspects of the self, writing your thoughts down without judgment or too much editing or analysis can be incredibly therapeutic. In the realm of digging up your past life memories, the journal is an invaluable tool that can assist you in getting things up and moving in the right direction.

I recommend you keep a journal specifically relating to this book and the material you're about to go through in the entirety of part 3. As we go along, you will be deepening your self- understanding and uncovering details about your soul journey that you will want to remember and build on as we go along. Without jotting these things down, you won't fully capture them all, so get a journal! You'll be so glad you did!

Back in the days before our fabulous phones and computers, I always kept a paper journal. I actually had to write my thoughts down with a pen! Amazing, right? These days, writing your thoughts down can come in many forms. You could do what I do and purchase a paper journal with a beautiful cover that you can keep and treasure for years to come. You could simply get a spiral notebook and jot thoughts down that way, or you can write in your computer, iPad, or even on an app in your phone. Either way, the process will help your conscious mind come into greater alignment with the thoughts that are deeply embedded in your memory from not only earlier in your current life, but in your past lives as well.

Every person has two aspects to their minds—their conscious mind, meaning the things that are happening in the present moment, and subconscious mind, which includes those things outside of conscious awareness. Everything you've ever done, seen, or experienced throughout the ages is stored in your subconscious mind. I like to think of the mind as a computer. You have all the documents at your disposal at any given time. Some documents you've opened up, and others are stored, just waiting to be accessed. By asking the right questions, deeply embedded memories can begin to emerge to support your healing journey. This chapter will take you through several exercises where I will guide you into spaces to allow these thoughts and feelings to surface and flow freely so that as we go along, you will receive more insights into your soul.

First up, let's get into the habit of writing these thoughts down. Find a journal, an app, or whatever makes you the most comfortable, and start the process. You may want to pick a favorite place to sit where you won't be disturbed. Play your favorite music and enjoy a cup of tea, wrap yourself up in a comfortable blanket, or do anything else that makes you feel comfortable and nurtured as you begin the process of revealing the deeper aspects of the soul.

This process should be as unconscious as possible—don't think or concentrate too much. Just allow thoughts and ideas to flow freely. Ready? Let's get started!

EXERCISE

Find a comfortable space where you can sit undisturbed for a few minutes. Pull out your tools that you will use to write, and just allow your mind to freely flow with anything you need to explore at this moment in time. Ask yourself this: *How do I feel right now?*

What thoughts bubble up as you contemplate the idea of uncovering some of your past life loves and other memories that may not be quite so pleasant?

What areas of the world come up when you think about places you either enjoyed visiting or would like to visit in the future?

What places do you dream about going to someday?

Which areas fascinated you to the point of watching shows about them on television?

After viewing documentaries or programming, what new places came into your awareness that struck a familiar feeling within you?

Think of any collections you have—knickknacks, art, decorations. Where are they from?

How did these items first come into your awareness?

What items are you drawn to that you may or may not collect right now?

Do you know the reason why you resonate with those things, or did the attraction bubble up out of nowhere?

Where did you go when you weren't having such a good time?

Have you ever had strange feelings in museums?

Are you drawn to gems and minerals? If so, which ones?

Are you repelled by any gems, stones, or other objects?

Have you ever met someone you felt you've known your whole life?

Did you ever encounter a person whom you immediately disliked even though you barely spoke to them?

Continue your freeform exercise and just allow yourself to write about anything and everything that comes up. Remember, this is not a thinking exercise. It's best, believe it or not, if you allow thoughts to float randomly and without judgment. Take your time and keep these notes so you can refer to them later. You may be surprised by what comes up!

Another tip is to keep the journal handy near your bedside. The subconscious thoughts, feelings, and memories that emerge during this process will continue to work themselves out in the dream state, so often when you are just waking up, you may find that answers to questions you've asked yourself are right in your mind, resolved, the moment you awaken. Keeping track of those ideas in the morning can be hugely beneficial. Great job!

Creating Your Life List

I'll tell you something about myself that you will probably find quite surprising. Although I love past lives and exploring those memories, I do not like exploring the earlier memories in my current life. Some of my life has been quite amazing, and other times have been quite challenging. You may know what I mean. I am a perpetual optimist, and I always look forward rather than back.

Despite that, healing involves bravely looking into the past, be it pleasant or unpleasant. There have been periods of my life that I choose to forget altogether and other times that I recall clear as a bell. During the years I struggled with stage four endometriosis, for example, I suffered through terrible pain and the loneliness of isolation, and those years can be super hard to recall. Those are definitely times I'd sooner forget.

Sometimes I've found it's important and even necessary to recall when certain major life events happened to gain perspective. One helpful exercise I do periodically is review those major milestones from time to time to see how I'm doing on the journey through life. To help myself easily recall such events, I created something called my Life List. I've found this tool so incredibly helpful, I want to share it with you here in case you'd like to do this yourself.

EXERCISE

As with many of the exercises in this section, go to your safe and comfortable space, put on some nice music, and pull out your journal, or do what I do and create a new document where you can write down these events.

Make a list of years beginning with the year of your birth, like this:

1980 (or whatever year)—born in XXX (list the city where you were born)

1982—sibling born (for example)

1990—moved to XXX

And so forth until you reach the current year.

You don't have to write down every single event, but list the highlights, such as the birth of siblings, switching schools, moving, taking trips—anything that seems important and is fresh on the top of your mind and in your easy-to-recall memories.

Once you make the list of the bigger-picture items, go through the list again. Write down where you worked and what year you started or left a particular company. This is a great exercise you need to do anyhow if you ever plan to apply for a job. On that note, to uncover those details, you could pull out your résumé and glean the information that way. Ask yourself these questions:

When did you start working at a particular place? When did you leave the company? What years did you attend high school and where did you go? What about college or any special classes you took? Think of sports you played, instruments you played, hobbies, clubs you participated in, and anything else you can recall. Did you sing in the church choir? When? Did you take road trips with your school to perform or play sports when you were younger?

Fill in those blanks, then think of other memories to add, such as years when loved ones passed or a time when you had a major life event that affected you profoundly. Put those all in the list and write them in order to gain the perspective of when those things occurred alongside other life events.

Once you've got the list, I recommend updating the list annually or semiannually. My list is done in a Word document, so about every six months, I go in and write down new items, then I save the document and rename it using the following format:

My Life List (Updated July 2020)

December or January is typically when I will go through that again, and once I briefly record a few highlights from the second half of this year, I will go in and rename it:

My Life List (Updated January 2021)

This is not easy to do at first, but once the main part is finished, it only takes five minutes or so to hit the highlights of a particular year. Here's an example of my life list for this year:

2020

January: traveled to Virginia Beach to teach a class

February: *Meet Your Karma* release and book signing

March: COVID shuts down the government

April: started teaching online via Zoom

May: *Past Lives with Pets* release and virtual book launch

June: participated in a virtual online conference with Llewellyn

You get the point. I don't mention much, but I include just enough details to trigger my memory for later when I may need to recall certain things about what happened. I don't usually get too emotional about these details. The goal is to simply recall things in the future when I might need to gain a broader perspective about the bigger picture or create more emotional writing in other places.

Your Life List may be more or less detailed than mine, and that's fine. Life is filled with ups and downs at times, and some years are far more emotional and challenging than others. You may have a lot to include in your list, or if you've had events you'd rather forget, you might choose to leave portions of your year blank. That's entirely up to you. The purpose of the Life List is to simply provide yourself with context you can use down the road of life.

Back in the day, I wanted my whole life to be filled with hearts and flowers, so to speak. As I get older, I see that recalling both pleasant and unpleasant things is very valuable as we go through the life journey. I've had a ton of huge blessings in addition to the challenges, and one thing I've learned over the years is that we need to express gratitude in our lives so we have more to be grateful for in the future.

Overall, I think that remembering your history is incredibly important to creating an amazing future. If you're like me, even though there are parts of the year you may not want to recall, sometime down the road, seeing all you've been through will make you realize how strong you are, and you will be amazed by all the challenges you've overcome. Enduring tough times creates a greater sense of gratitude when things are going well. In the end, it's all up to you.

Life is full of contrasting experiences. When we embrace them all and go forward, we start to understand that we carry the strength within to withstand any challenge. I hope this idea of a Life List will help you move forward into the life you truly want to live.

Remembering Trips from the Past

To get you ready to go into past lives, we need to do some preparation to dig into your memories so you will be able to find the situations that most need healing or that would be most helpful and revealing to you on your life journey. This short exercise will help you take a trip down memory lane to specifically recall the trips you loved the most. Ready? Let's begin!

EXERCISE

If possible, pull out your old photo albums or computer files where you keep photos. Take your time gathering up what you can.

Once you've found all you can, sit in your comfortable space where you were before. Prepare yourself with music and other comfort items, including blankets, pillows, and any drinks or snacks that make you feel supported. Pull your journal out as you prepare to consider the following questions. Ask yourself the following:

What photos did you uncover? What were you doing and where did you go? Look at the photos. How do you look? Happy? Upset? Allow yourself to recall anything about those trips and make any notes that may be helpful to you later on down the road.

If you're like me, you may not remember much about the past. That's fine. Just gaze at the photos and allow yourself to form the first impression that comes to your mind. Do you think the people in the photos are having fun or not? Which trips emerge as your favorites? Which ones were not so pleasant and why? Make a list and consider notating whether your trip turned out pleasant, horrible, uneventful, or anything in between. Very good.

Once you've gone through the photos you still have, you may realize there were trips you did not photograph, or the pictures may have been lost through the years. Go ahead and think back through your life. Imagine you can travel back into your memories to the earliest time you can that may not be in your photos. What's the earliest trip you can recall taking?

Where did you go? Whom did you go with? How did you feel there? Allow yourself to recall anything you can about the experience. Did you like this location or not? Why?

From that early time in your current life history, imagine you can move forward toward now. Imagine you can easily recall other trips you took over the years, and make a list of whatever comes up. As with all exercises, don't think too much. Gain the impression of how you felt, good or bad, and allow those feelings to be what they are without attempting to judge or change anything. Know that all is well.

These processes are theoretically easy, but they take time. You may need to do this in several different sittings in order to go through every single event, or you may only want to recall the highlights. Either way, taking that trip down memory lane will help you uncover the memories of the times you loved and enjoyed and make room for healing and transformation of events that were more challenging, which will ultimately make you a happier you.

Expanding Awareness of a Favorite Place

Now that you've been digging up so much from the past, you've undoubtedly uncovered a few places you love. We have so many experiences in our lives that sometimes it's hard to keep track of them, even when they're pleasant. Between your Life List and the process of digging through your old pictures, you should have at least a few places in mind that you really loved and had a chance to recall some cherished memories.

A great place to begin your exploration of Supretrovie is by going back in time and deeply tuning in to a happy memory from one of the trips you took. Chances are good that you loved those places for a reason that goes beyond your current lifetime. Let's take another short trip in your mind to locate a memory of one of your special places. For this exercise, you will be closing your eyes, so you may want to read to yourself in your recording app so you can play the audio back anytime. Ready? Great!

EXERCISE

Sit in your comfortable place with your feet flat on the floor and your hands in your lap and close your eyes. Take a deep, healing breath in through your nose, and exhale out your mouth. Relax. Allow your mind to go back to one of the favorite places you recalled during your recent trips down memory lane. You may have found more than one, so allow your Higher Self to notice the first place that floats into your mind. Very good.

Think about that place now. What did you love about it? Imagine you can recall the pictures, thoughts, and feelings you had while you were there. Take your time and notice what you notice.

[PAUSE]

As you reflect on this incredibly pleasant time, what is the most important thing you learned or gained from your trip to this favorite place? How is this influencing your life? Very good.

When I count back from three, you will open your eyes and come back into the room, feeling awake, refreshed, and better than you felt before. Ready? Three, grounded, centered, and balanced; two, still considering this place in your dreams tonight, so by tomorrow morning, you may have new insights into this place that you can easily include in your journal writings; and one, you're back!

How did that go? Remember, you could do this exercise for any of your favorite places so you can receive insights into how those journeys affected your life. Good job!

Expanding Awareness of a Least Favorite or Unpleasant Place

If you love a place, there's a connection to explore. Unfortunately, the same holds true if you're not as excited about a particular location. I know that firsthand! In this next journey, you will safely and gently tap into a less amazing memory so you can find the places where your past life journeys can provide the most healing. Ready to take a look? Good job!

EXERCISE

Sit in your comfortable place with your feet flat on the floor and your hands in your lap and close your eyes. Take a deep, healing breath in through your nose, and exhale out your mouth. Relax. Allow your mind to go back to one of the unpleasant places you recalled during your recent trips down memory lane. You may have found more than one, so allow your Higher Self to notice the first place that floats into your mind. Very good.

Think about that place now. What did you dislike about that place? Imagine you can recall the pictures, thoughts, and feelings you had while you were there. Take your time and notice what you notice.

[PAUSE]

As you reflect on this unpleasant experience, what is the most important thing you learned during your journey? Notice what you notice. How is this influencing your life to this day? Very good.

When I count back from three, you will open your eyes and come back into the room, feeling awake, refreshed, and better than you felt before. Ready? Three, grounded, centered, and balanced; two, processing the learning in your dreams tonight, so by tomorrow morning, you are fully integrated into this new energy and can easily include new insights in your journal that will help you on your life path; and one, you're back!

How did you do? What's interesting is the fact that our most challenging times can eventually become our greatest gifts in life. You can gain incredibly valuable lessons that you can carry forward throughout your life journey to make your life healthier, happier, and more peaceful because of the lessons received early on.

I challenge you to look at all the more difficult memories in this way by tuning in and embracing the journey as you go. Great job!

Tuning In to Pleasant Memories from Your Past

You don't have to travel around the world to experience Supretrovie. In this next process, you will tap into more happy memories that emerge from your subconscious mind. This may provide further areas of exploration for the regressions you'll do in an upcoming chapter. Even the simplest things that bring you the most joy can be reminiscent of a past life memory. Ready to find out? Wonderful!

EXERCISE

Sit in your comfortable space, close your eyes, and relax. Take a deep, healing breath in through your nose and exhale. Breathe in peace and tranquility, exhale any tensions. Very good.

Allow a healing white light to move from head to toe, cleansing away any unwanted energies and making you feel more and more relaxed. Notice now that the light begins to move through your heart center, forming a protective shield of golden light that surrounds you by about three feet in all directions. Feel yourself floating inside the golden ball, safe and secure, noticing that within the golden light, only that which is of your highest good can come through.

There is a door in front of you. It may be a door you've walked through before. Go ahead now and walk or float through that door and find yourself inside your special space. Feel the loving energies there, and notice that your angel or guide has appeared to greet you.

Imagine your guide is sitting at a table and showing you a book. Take a seat and get comfortable as you flip through the book, through pleasant memories of your past. Imagine you can begin at the front of this book, flipping past early memories, times that made you feel happy and peaceful. Notice what you notice. What memories are emerging?

What were you doing in these happy times? Why did this moment emerge as so important to your life journey?

If needed, allow your guide to share any special information with you about these early times that would help you on your path.

[PAUSE]

Very good. Continue to flip through the pages, noticing anything else that you need to remember today about happy times from the past.

[PAUSE]

When you're ready, close the book. Thank your guide for assisting you today. Stand up and walk or float back toward the door where you came in and go through the door now, closing it behind you.

When I count back from five, you will return, feeling awake, refreshed, and better than you felt before. Ready? Five, grounded, centered, and balanced; four, recalling these happy times further in your dreams tonight, so by tomorrow morning, you will remember those fun times and allow those happy memories to help you create an amazing new day for yourself; three, driving and being safe in all activities; two, grounded, centered, and balanced; and one, you're back!

Did you find some happy times? Did anything unexpected emerge? Hopefully recalling those good times will help you create more fun energy in the future and will assist you as you continue to tap into your past from both your current lifetime as well as later on when we go into your past incarnations. Great job!

Healing & Cutting Cords with Unpleasant Memories

Along the same lines as the last exercise, this time, you will allow your Higher Self and subconscious mind to present you with any unpleasant memory. Your bigger intention is to use this information later down the road, and I think you'll be surprised how an unpleasant memory that you may have completely forgotten about could provide you with a deep healing later in the book. Let's take a look and see what emerges. Ready? Great!

EXERCISE

Sit in your safe space, close your eyes, and allow yourself to relax as you once again bring a protective shield of golden light around you. This ball of light is surrounding you now by three feet or more in all directions. Know that you are safe and protected within this light.

Walk or float through the door. Once again, you will find your guide waiting with a book for you to examine. Feel the loving and supportive energy of your guide as you open the book and leaf through the pages to an unpleasant memory.

Notice what you notice, and as you do, you will see, feel, or imagine a cord of white light coming out of your solar plexus (stomach area) and connecting you with the event you're seeing within the book. Imagine that your guide has a pair of golden scissors. When I count to three, your guide will cut the cord between you and this memory. Ready? One, two, three—cutting that cord now.

As your guide cuts the cord, a stunning white healing light is coming down from above, moving through this cut cord, traveling into your stomach, your heart, your legs and feet, and up through your arms, neck, and shoulders and into your mind. Imagine the light getting brighter and brighter, lighter and lighter, healing you and releasing any negative energy from those unpleasant events. Take your time and allow this light to work until you feel completely relaxed.

[PAUSE]

When you're ready, close the book. If you need any additional information or assistance from your guide, go ahead and receive that now.

[PAUSE]

Very good. Thank your guide for helping you with this healing today and walk back through the door where you came in, closing that door behind you.

In a moment, when I count back from five, you will be back, feeling awake, refreshed, and better than you felt before. Ready? Five, grounded, centered, and balanced; four, allowing the healing light you received to continue to lift your spirits throughout the rest of today and overnight, so by tomorrow, you will feel lighter and happier than ever before; three, always being safe in everything you do; two, grounded, centered, and balanced; and one, you're back!

Wonderful work! Cord cutting is such a powerful process to help you release unwanted energy and disconnect with anything you need to heal at any time. Use this process often to lighten and brighten your day!

Psychometry with an Object

Earlier, we did an exercise to cut the energetic cords between you and any unpleasant memories. Cord cutting is always a great tool to keep with you during the life journey because that visualization can transmute unwanted influences easily and quickly.

But what happens if you actually want to connect with something outside of yourself, such as an object? You can use the power of psychic sensing, also known as psychometry, to consciously follow those cords of light back to the origin points of objects so you can learn more about them.

In this next exercise, you're going to hold an object and do your best to tune in without overthinking. There's always that temptation to say, "It feels like I'm making this up, but ..." and if you feel that way, wonderful! Just don't let those thoughts stop you from completing your task and receiving the information your object wants to tell you.

In reality, every single thing in this universe is made up of energy. Physical objects are no different. We can all pick up feelings from things if we take a moment to quiet the conscious mind and listen to what things are trying to tell us.

Ideally, you would practice with another person who gives you an object that you're not familiar with, but you can also do this exercise on your own with anything you have lying around. To get started, I suggest you pick out something from your home. It could be an item you love, or anything you feel drawn to at this moment. Choose an object you enjoy first, then do the exercise again and try tuning in to something you're not as fond of to see what happens. Once you find what you're looking for, settle in, and let's get you ready for the exploration.

Like all the exercises in this book, you may want to record this and play it back to yourself so you can concentrate on what's happening and do the journey again at a later time. Ready? Let's begin.

EXERCISE

Select any object you're guided to use for this process. Sit in your familiar and comfortable meditation space. You may enjoy quiet healing music, or you may find it easier to be quiet so you can hear any guidance received. Hold the object in your hands and close your eyes. If the object is too large for that, sit near it with your palms pressed on the item and close your eyes. Very good.

While holding the object, breathe in peace, relaxation, and healing, and exhale any tensions. Imagine you can clear your mind and focus solely on the object. Feel how it feels in your hand. Is it heavy? Light? Hard? Soft? Fluffy? Notice what you notice.

Next, imagine there is a beam of light that comes out of that object and floats away from it. Take your consciousness now and follow that line of light. Float out along the line and imagine this line of light going all the way back to the place where the object originated from.

Notice pictures, thoughts, and feelings that emerge. Don't judge anything. Simply see what you see. Do you notice any people? Places? More importantly, how does the object feel? Imagine it's easy to notice what feelings come up as you tune in. Once you notice the predominant feeling, where did that feeling come from? A prior owner? A creator or artisan who crafted the object? The factory where the item was manufactured? Allow any thoughts to bubble up in your mind.

If necessary, imagine you can now close this energy off. If needed, go ahead and cut the cord between you and the object and disconnect from that energy. Ready? Three, two, one—cutting the cord. Send a beautiful healing light around the object and around yourself. See this light bringing you joy, peace, harmony, and happiness. When you're ready, open your eyes, feeling awake, refreshed, and better than you felt before. Very good!

How did you do? You may want to take note of anything interesting that came up. Were you surprised? Later in the book, we will do a past life regression dealing with an object that fascinates you so you can learn more. For now, I suggest practicing this process, and know you can get better at it over time. Great job!

Artifact or Antique Exercise

Older items can often have lingering energies from prior situations or owners. This happens because, believe it or not, thoughts are things. The energetic residue from times long gone lingers on everything, and the energy is especially strong with ancient artifacts or antiques in general.

If you're a super sensitive person, tuning in to the energy around older items can be easy. For others, you may have to practice a bit. Still, anyone can learn to tune in with a little practice. This next exercise will help you do just that.

Before you begin, select the item you're curious about. If you can hold it in your hand, that's great. If it's larger, then do this next exercise in such a way that you can touch it if you can. If neither option is possible—for example, if you saw something in a museum that affected you—then you can still do this process using your imagination. Ideally, you'll be able to use your sense of touch to go deeper into the energy. Ready?

EXERCISE

Sit in your comfortable spot and hold the artifact or antique you want to learn about. Imagine you can follow an invisible line of light that connects the item to the past. Allow any pictures, thoughts, impressions, or feelings to come through.

How do you feel holding or touching this item? What impressions are you having? Do you see people? Places? Allow anything and everything to float into your mind without judgment.

Take your time. Notice what you notice. Once these impressions begin to slow down, imagine you can close off that energy and surround yourself and the artifact in a ball of protective light. When you're ready, open your eyes and come back into the room.

Great job! Write any important information down in your journal for future reference and keep practicing! You'll definitely get better and better over time.

Cutting Cords with Artifacts, Objects, or Gemstones to Clear Unwanted Influences

Anytime you're dealing with old objects, antiques, or artifacts, because everything in the universe is made up of energy, you may pick up vibes along the way. Hopefully the energy is good, but if it's not, you can always cut the cords.

Cord cutting is an amazing and easy thing to do to cleanse things when you first purchase them or to clear out any unwanted energy you pick up while working with or being in the presence of various things you encounter in life. For highly sensitive people, it's a good idea to get in the practice of cutting cords anytime you acquire new things because everything picks up energy from the store where you purchased it, from the supply chain, and from the manufacturer. A simple ritual can help you connect to your new purchase with ease and clarity.

EXERCISE

Select any object you'd like to clear. Sit with the object in a comfortable chair. Imagine there's an energetic cord connecting the object to the outer world. Use your inner vision to imagine a pair of golden scissors emerging so you can easily cut the cords between your item and the outer world. Imagine this cord is connected to all people, places, and things associated with the object in the past. To clear the object, imagine you can cut cords between your object and all prior owners or origins. In a moment, you can cut that cord, clearing all the energy and neutralizing the object. Ready? Three, two, one, and cut! Imagine the golden scissors cutting the light cord and a beautiful healing light pouring down over you and your object, removing any unwanted energies. When you're ready, open your eyes and come back into the room, feeling awake, refreshed, and better than you did before.

Connecting Your Energy to an Object

Once the cords are cut between your new stuff and the outer world, you can also consciously make a divine connection to your new item so the two of you will have a wonderfully balanced and productive relationship. Ready?

EXERCISE

Still holding the object of your choice, go through the previous exercise and cut cords between your new item and the outer world. Very good. When you're ready, you can imagine there is a beautiful string of bright white light coming out of your stomach or solar plexus area and connecting you with the new item. Imagine you can connect this cord as the new owner and send a loving, peaceful energy to the object, knowing that you will now be able to fully use and connect with this item in the highest way possible.

If guided, you may ask the object questions:

• How can we best work together?
• What would you enjoy doing most?
• Any special things I should know about you?

Imagine the item can share any insights in making this a harmonious relationship. Imagine a stunning healing light surrounding the two of you, and know that only that which is of your highest good can come through. Thank your new item for assisting you and know you can now enjoy a long and productive partnership. When you're ready, open your eyes and come back into the room.

When you really think of it, objects are part of this universe, so why not attempt to get into better energetic rapport with them? I know this works especially well with electronics. No sense to get upset and yell at your computer, for example, because that can actually make the situation worse. It's best to arrange an easy journey in advance and then watch as your intentions manifest themselves in the physical world.

Reading a Gemstone

In a similar fashion to how you would tune in to any object of interest, reading the impressions from a gemstone can be quite interesting. For this next exercise, ideally you will have a gem or stone to hold. The stone doesn't need to be anything fancy or special. Just use whatever you're guided to practice on. You're going to dig deeper in this process because there are many areas and energies you might pick up—everything from the country where your gem is from, to the mine itself, to many of the people who transported the stone to the place you found it. Be open and see what happens. Ready? Great! Let's get started!

EXERCISE

Sit in a comfortable space with your stone or gem in your hands. Close your eyes and breathe. Place your gem directly in the center of your palms and press your palms together. Notice how you can feel the energy of this stone. Continue to breathe as you bring a pure white light down from head to toe. Allow the light to relax you and clear your energy field in preparation for your journey today.

When I count to three, you will be clear and prepared. Ready? One, two, and three. You're clear! Be cleared of any residual energy now and once again tune in to the feeling of the stone pressed in your palms. Very good.

Imagine that stone is becoming lighter and lighter, brighter and brighter. Notice as this stone lights up; there's a beam of light emanating out of the stone, and that ray of light is moving off into the distance. Use your mind to trace that line of light as it moves from your stone and travels back in time to the source of this stone, to the first place where this stone was found.

When I count to three, you will arrive at this earliest moment. Ready? One, two, and three. Be there now. Feel the energy of this earliest occurrence. See what you see, or hear any information that may float into your mind. Where is this place? How does this feel? What time frame is this?

If you don't know, imagine a geological period emerging in your mind. Very good. Ask the stone, "Is this the earliest time I can experience with you today?" Notice if you get a yes or a no. Trust the answer. If yes, good job. If no, imagine you can go back further in time to the real source of this stone. Be there now. Notice what you notice.

Where in the world are you? What's happening? From this earliest moment, imagine you can fast-forward through major events in this stone's journey to you. Whom did this stone encounter? What part or parts of the world did this stone exist in? Notice workers, miners, prior owners. Take your time and observe any people, places, or feelings along the way. Allow that energy to bring you all the way up to the present moment. Be back in the present moment now.

Notice that you can cut the cord between this gem and all prior owners and situations. Notice that light cord, and in a moment, imagine a pair of golden scissors cutting the stone free from its past, clearing the way for a pure connection between the two of you. Ready? Three, two, one, and cut!

Feel the amazing energy as your stone gets lighter and brighter than ever before. Very nice. In a moment, when I count from three, you will come back into the room, feeling awake and refreshed. Three—grounded, centered, and balanced—two, and one. You're back!

How did that go? Were you able to travel to where your stone is from? Did you see any people along the way? Did the stone go to more than one country before coming to be with you? Nice!

Selecting a Gem or Stone

When gems come into your life, that connection happens for a reason. The consciousness of that exact mineral chose to be in your presence, or you are tapping into that energy for some higher purpose.

Collecting rocks as souvenirs can be quite tempting, and in some cases, you may be truly called to take some with you, whether shopping in a store or hiking in a natural setting. How will you decide which to take and which to leave behind? By quieting your mind and listening to them. Stones will talk to you if you have the patience to hear what they're saying. This isn't like having a conversation with a friend, mind you; it's more a thought that pops up out of nowhere.

This next exercise will give you the steps to connect with stones or any object you're considering buying to ensure doing so is for your highest good. Whether you're in a store or out in nature, follow these steps to select what gem, stone, or mineral is best for you to work with at any given time in your life. Ready? Great!

EXERCISE

1. Approach the stones either in the store or out in nature.

2. Put your hands out, palms facing the energy. Notice how this feels to you.

3. Notice a rock or stone that speaks to you by drawing your attention more than any of the other stones available. Again, notice how you feel with the stone.

4. If the feeling is good, reach down, pick it up, and hold the stone in your hand.

5. Allow the energy from the stone to affect you and work with your energy to make whatever adjustment is necessary.

6. Quiet your mind and listen. Focus all your energy and attention on that stone, then, either aloud or to yourself, ask, "Are you for me?" or, "Do you want to come home with me?"

7. Listen for an answer.

8. Notice the first answer that pops into your mind. Don't judge or edit. If it's a yes, continue on.

9. If the answer is no, place the stone back where you found it and move on.

10. Accept the answer you receive and either take the stone or move on to another.

Try this the next time you're having a hard time making a decision about which pieces to buy. If you need a more visual cue, you can also use a pendulum to decide which stone or object is for you. Ask the question and let the pendulum give you an answer for yes or no. Again, accept the results. If you are drawn to a stone or gem, there's no doubt that's happening for a reason. Who knows—perhaps the stone will help you heal a past life.

Tuning In to Your Soul—Anamnesis Exercise

Throughout this book, we've explored the idea that you may not actually need a past life regression to understand who you were in times long gone. In this next exercise, you will explore Plato's concept of anamnesis, or soul knowing.

According to Plato, your soul already knows who you were before and what you were doing in any prior lifetime. The challenge lies in the many distractions in our physical world that prevent us from automatically having that understanding without undergoing hypnosis. This process will expand your awareness and may give you some insightful information along the way.

EXERCISE

Sit in your chair with eyes closed, resting comfortably. Breathe in through your nose, exhale out your mouth, and notice that each breath makes you more and more relaxed.

Bringing that gorgeous healing white light down from above, notice how it washes from head to feet, moving through the crown of your head, down your spine, and into the soles of your feet. You are relaxed and healed. A beautiful ball of gold light surrounds you now. This light is protective, like a shield. Only that which is of your highest good can come through this light. Likewise, this light illuminates your soul knowing. Feel the light expand your energy field around your body so you feel connected to all time. Good job.

Now walk or float through your special door into your sacred space. As you go inside, your guide welcomes you and invites you to sit in a chair. Do that now. Sit and relax. Very nice.

Allow your mind to expand with each breath. With your guide's help, you expand your awareness out of your own physical body to the world around you and to all people, places, and things that have ever been or ever will be. As you do this, ask your guide to assist you in uncovering some of the lives you've lived in the past.

Who were you? Allow pictures, thoughts, and feelings to emerge. Your guide may also tell you any helpful details you need to make this information more readily available to you.

What parts of the world did you live in? Were you ever on planets other than Earth? Notice what you notice. See what you see and feel what you feel.

What is the most important past experience that you can draw upon right now to help you in your current lifetime? Allow a thought to bubble up into your mind. Very good. Why is that so important to you today in your present experience? Listen to the words or thoughts that come up when you ask that important question.

Take a moment and ask your guide for any clarity you may need. When you're ready, stand up and thank your guide. Turn and walk back through the door and go out to where you started.

In a moment, you will return to the present time, feeling more aware than ever before. Three, grounded, centered, and balanced; two, processing what you received in your dreams, so by tomorrow morning, new insights about these early times will be revealed; and one, you're back!

What did your soul tell you? Had you consciously thought about this before, or not? Could you see why that experience can help you now? With practice, this process can become easier over time. The truth is that you are more powerful than you give yourself credit for, so own your power, and know what you know! Great job!

Summing Up

Developing psychic awareness in ourselves can be so helpful in assisting us to better understand ourselves and the world around us. When you consciously tune in to objects, or even to the quietest parts of your soul and mind, you realize that we are more connected to all time—past, present, and future—than we may have ever thought possible. Extending love and light to all areas of our life can yield huge results on the path to wholeness and peace. I hope this section helped you make more room for happiness in your life.

Chapter Six

• • • •

PAST LIFE HEALING JOURNEYS

WE'VE FINALLY ARRIVED AT the section you've been waiting for—past life clearings. Once you uncover interesting places and things you have a connection to, the healing comes when you can deepen that experience and understanding by traveling into the specific areas in your former lifetimes where you lived or visited, or used and encountered various objects. I'll guide you through several ways you can experience real healing from the influences of Supretrovie by going through past life regressions to gather more information about why you were affected in various life situations. Let's get started!

Past Life Regression to a Favorite Place

Earlier in the book, you dug into your memories of places you visited in the past. Based on that, go ahead and think of your favorite place in the world. Hold that special place in your heart and mind as we explore your connection to that area in the context of your past lives and soul history.

Remember, this special place doesn't have to be anything exotic. You may be enthralled by a small town near your home or a specific neighborhood in your city. We've done so much exploring up to this point, so if you find yourself unable to pick just one place, know that you can definitely do this journey over again with each favorite place you'd like to explore. I recommend beginning with the first place that floats into your mind. Ready? Let's begin.

EXERCISE

Sit in a comfortable place with your feet flat on the floor and your hands in your lap. Close your eyes. Breathe in peace and healing and relaxation, and exhale any tensions and concerns. Very good.

With each breath you take, you're becoming more and more relaxed. Imagine now there's a beam of pure white light coming down through the top of your head, moving through your head, neck, and shoulders, down into your arms, wrists, hands, and fingers. The light is flowing down your spine, relaxing and healing you as it moves through your heart and stomach, into your legs, your knees, ankles, and all the way down into the soles of your feet. Allow this light to pour through you from head to toe, removing any tensions and concerns as you send unwanted energy into the earth where it is transformed into a healing, loving light. Very good.

The light is becoming stronger now, so strong it begins to pour from your heart, creating a beautiful golden ball of light that surrounds you by about three feet in all directions. Feel yourself floating in the golden light, safe, secure, and totally carefree, knowing that within this golden ball of light, only that which is of your highest good can come through. Very good.

Imagine there's a doorway in front of you. You can either see the door, feel the door, or just know the door is there. In a moment, when I count to three, you will open that door and step inside a safe and sacred space. Ready? One, two, three; open the door. Walk inside the beautiful room where you feel safe, secure, and protected. Very good.

Imagine you can look around this room. Notice what's there. Feel the peaceful vibrations of this sacred space and know that you are totally safe, secure, and relaxed. Very good.

As you take a look around, notice that a beautiful angel or spirit guide is floating down in front of you. Imagine they can be there now, this special guide who knows everything there is to know about you, your soul, and your soul's journey. Feel the deep sense of unconditional love and high regard your angel has for you. Your guide has come here today to assist you in uncovering some very important things about yourself.

Go ahead now and take your guide by the hand. The two of you will begin to float. You're floating up, up, up, out of the room, floating higher and higher and higher, up, up, up and into the clouds. Notice that the higher up you float, the more relaxed you feel.

You and your guide have floated so high in the sky that as you look down, you notice a ray of sunshine below you. You're floating over today, and in a moment, your guide will help you float back to a very early time—to the source event, the real source of your connection to the favorite place you're asking about today.

When I count to three, you will float back to that source event. Ready? One, floating back, back, back; two, further

and further, going way, way, way back to the real source of
your connection to your favorite place; and three. Be there
now, floating over that event. Imagine you can hold your
guide's hand and float down, down, down into that event. Be
there now. Notice what's happening.

Where are you? Notice the first thing that comes to your
mind. What year is it? How do you feel? Are you a man or
woman? Are you alone or with other people? Take a moment
and notice all you can.

[PAUSE]

Go ahead now and float into the next most significant
event in this lifetime where you're with other people. Be
there now. What's happening? Who are you with? What's
your relationship to them? As you experience the energy of
the people around you, is there anyone there you know in
your current life? Maybe, maybe not. Notice if anyone feels
familiar to you. If so, who are they? How is the relationship
you had back then similar to the things you're experiencing
together in your current life? Very good.

What's happening in this very early time? Why are these
events significant to your soul journey?

[PAUSE]

Continue to move through the major events of that life you
lived in one of your favorite places. Notice what you notice, see
what you see, feel what you feel.

[PAUSE]

Remember you are still surrounded by a golden ball of
light. Know that within this golden ball of light, you are safe,
secure, protected. Go ahead now and fast-forward to the
very last day of your life in this wonderful place. Be there
now. Notice how you pass into spirit. Go ahead and do that

now. Feel yourself lifting up, up, up, out of that body, out of that life.

Float into the peaceful space between lives. Be there now, with your loving guide. As you recall the life you just visited, what lessons did you learn during that important time in your soul's history? How are those lessons affecting you in your current incarnation?

Thinking about this place you love, why did your soul go back there in your current life? What purpose did that serve?

[PAUSE]

Very good. Now, take all the energy you need from this experience, and imagine you can take your guide by the hand, and the two of you will begin floating down, down, down, back through the clouds, down, down, down, back into the beautiful room where we started. Be there now, inside the beautiful room.

Take a moment and ask your guide for any other helpful information you need at this moment. If you have questions, ask your guide to clarify anything you need to better understand.

[PAUSE]

Very good. Thank your guide for joining you today. Imagine they can float away. Now turn and walk or float back toward the doorway you first entered. Go ahead and walk or float through that door and go back out to the place where we started. Close the door behind you and know that you will return to this place soon. Very good.

You're still surrounded by golden light, safe and secure. When I count down from five, you will return to the room, feeling awake, refreshed, and better than you felt before. Ready?

Five, grounded, centered, and balanced; four, continuing to process this information in your dreams tonight, so by tomorrow morning, you will be fully integrated into this new information; three, driving safely and being safe in all activities; two, grounded, centered, and balanced; and one, you're back!

How did you do? Were you surprised by what you discovered? Why did you return in your current life to that place? You will probably want to explore this in your journal. I recommend writing down any insights from this journey and keeping track of that as we go forward. Remember also that you can go back and repeat this or any of the regressions to gain more insights and important information that will help you on your life path. Great job!

Past Life Regression & Healing for an Unpleasant Place

Personally, I am not a huge fan of reviewing unpleasant memories. Then again, who is? Still, what I've found over the years is that doing so can make more room for peace and happiness in my life experience. This has also been the case for my clients, and I truly believe the same can happen for you. When you're ready to challenge yourself, pull out your notes and review the thoughts and feelings you had about the places you despised or areas where you had a less-than-optimal experience. Again, I'd go with the first location that emerges. Your soul knows what's best for your highest purpose at any given time. When you've got that place firmly in your mind's eye, settle in and go on the following journey.

EXERCISE

Sit in your comfortable space. Take a deep, healing breath in through your nose, exhaling out your mouth. Close your eyes and relax. Imagine a beautiful beam of pure white light moving down through the top of your head, through your face, your jaw, moving into your neck and shoulders. The light flows down your arms and into your wrists, hands, and fingers. Feel the loving energy of this light moving into your heart and stomach as it makes its way down the body into your legs and moves all the way down into your feet.

Allow this light to wash away any tensions as it pours out of your heart, surrounding you with a protective ball of healing golden light that measures about three feet in all directions. Know that within this golden light, only that which is of your highest good can come through.

Notice now there is a doorway in front of you. This is the same door you've seen before, so it feels totally safe and familiar. Know that this door leads to your sacred safe place. Open the door now and walk or float inside this beautiful space. Be there now. Notice that your guide, whom you've met before, is with you now, saying hello.

Feel the unconditional love this guide has for you. Know that your guide is here to assist you with a special healing today concerning a place where you've been in the past. Take your guide by the hand as the two of you begin to float. Lifting up, up, up off the ground, you find yourselves floating higher and higher and higher. Know that the higher up you float, the more relaxed you feel. Floating out the ceiling of the beautiful room, you and your guide are in the clouds, peaceful and so very relaxed. Up, up, up, you float away, into those clouds, until you find yourself so high in the sky that you notice a ray of sunshine below you. Imagine this ray of light represents time, and you and your loving guide are gently floating over the present day. Very good. Notice now that you can turn your attention in the direction of your past.

In just a moment, you will both begin to float back over the past to the real source event, to the earliest time when you first encountered the place you're thinking about today.

You are asking your guide to assist you in learning the real reason why that particular area is troubling to you, knowing you are still surrounded by the golden light and that only that which is of your highest good will come through. Ready? Floating back, over your past. Further and further back. When I count to three, you will arrive at this very early time in your soul's history, the source event or the most important event that will best explain your reaction to this place in your current life. Ready? One, floating back in time; two, further and further; and three. You're there. Be there now. Imagine you can float down, down, down into that event. Notice what's happening.

Where are you? Note the first thing that comes to your mind. What year is this? Are you alone or with other people? If so, who are they? Does anyone seem familiar? Take a moment now to notice all you can. Very good. If needed, imagine you can ask your guide to explain anything you need to clarify.

[PAUSE]

Imagine next that you can fast-forward to the next most significant event in that lifetime where you are with other people. Be there now. Notice what's happening. What are the dynamics between you and the other people? Fast-forward through other major events. Notice what you notice. Feel what you feel. Allow your Higher Self and soul to go right into the event that caused you to dislike this place. Be there now. What's happening? Very good.

Now, lift out of those events; go higher and higher and higher. Float above those challenging times. Allow your guide to send a healing, loving light down to everyone involved in this situation. Imagine the light is transforming everyone, healing them all, and neutralizing these negative feelings. Take your time until this situation feels better.

[PAUSE]

Notice there is an energetic cord of light that is connecting you with the events below. That light is coming out of your stomach or solar plexus area and connecting you with the person you used to be. Notice now that your guide has a big pair of golden scissors. When I count to three, your guide will cut the cord between you and these events, releasing you from any unwanted influences. Ready? One, two, three, and cut! Allow a stunning white light to flow from above, healing everyone in this early time. That light is now flowing into that cut cord, and it moves into your stomach, heart, and lungs. It's moving through your legs, feet, arms, hands, and up, up, up into your neck and shoulders, into your head and mind. Feel the light heal you and release you from any heavy energy. Notice that you feel lighter and brighter than before. Very good!

Now imagine as you and your loving guide float over this very early time. Thanks to this new, more neutral energy, you can understand some important things about these events. What lessons did you learn there? How do these lessons apply to things you're going through in your current lifetime? Why did your soul choose to consciously return to this place in your present incarnation? What did you learn by doing so? Take your time to find answers.

[PAUSE]

While your guide continues to send this healing light to all involved, imagine there's another energetic cord connecting you with the situation, the other people involved, and the actual events. Your guide brings out the pair of golden scissors again. In a moment, when I count to three, your guide will cut the cord between you and these events, freeing you from any unwanted influences. Ready? One, two, three, and cut! Feel another bright healing light coming down from above begin to merge into this cut cord. That light travels into your stomach and heart, through your neck and shoulders, into your mind, then down through your legs and feet. The light is healing and relaxing you, making you feel better than ever before as it releases you energetically from all other people and the event itself. Beginning right now, you are no longer affected by these events in your current lifetime. Very good.

Allow that loving light to lift you higher and higher and higher, above these events as you float into the beautiful space between lives. Take your guide's hand as the two of you begin to float back, down, down, down, back through the clouds, until you land in the safe space where we began. Be there now, feeling better than before. Very nice!

Thank your guide for helping you today as they float away. Turn and walk back through the door where you started, closing it behind you. Go back out to that space and prepare to return. Ready?

Five, processing all the healing received in your dreams, so by tomorrow, you will be fully integrated into this new energy and information; four, driving safely, being safe in all activities; three, grounded, centered, and balanced; two, feeling lighter and brighter than ever before; one, and you're back!

How did you enjoy that? Do you feel lighter as a result of this healing? I hope so! Again, I encourage you to make notes in your journal of significant thoughts or feelings that will help you as we go along. No doubt, you may experience dreams about this experience or any of the exercises in this section, so you may also want to keep the journal near your nightstand so you can jot down any thoughts or ideas that come in overnight that may be helpful to your soul journey. I applaud you for taking a deeper look at the less-than-pleasant things from the past. Doing so can yield amazing results for you as you bring more light and peace into your daily experience. Great work!

Past Life Regression to the Source Event with an Object

Next up, we're going to take you on a journey to explore the deeper mysteries behind your connection to an object. People are drawn to objects for a reason, so think about something you've been attracted to in the past. It may be the same object you chose for our earlier exercise in psychometry.

If possible, you could hold the object you're attracted to while you go through this experience, because there's no doubt that would enhance the experience, but if you don't currently own the object, or if it's something you saw in a store or elsewhere, then no worries. Either way, you're going to find helpful answers.

During this regression, you'll have a chance to deepen your understanding of why you like certain things, and what you may find is that you're drawn to familiar items from your past. Learning more about yourself and coming to a greater understanding about the complexities of your soul will pay off big-time later in life. You will learn to have newfound love and respect for the most important person in your life—yourself. Get ready to settle in, and let's get started!

EXERCISE

Sit in your familiar, comfortable space. Close your eyes and breathe. Inhale joy and peace and harmony, and exhale tensions and concerns. Very good. Imagine a beam of pure white light moving from head to feet, relaxing and healing you. Allow that light to easily pour from your heart center, creating that beautiful golden ball of light that surrounds you by about three feet in all directions. Allow yourself to float peacefully inside the protective shield of golden light, knowing only that which is of your highest good can come through.

Notice the doorway in front of you, the door you've been through before. Open that door now and walk inside your sacred space. Your guide is there. Say hello. Take your guide's hand and begin to float away, up through the ceiling. Floating higher and higher up into the clouds. The higher up you float, the more relaxed you feel.

You and your guide are now floating so high in the sky, you find yourselves floating over today. Ask your guide an important question: Why am I so attracted to this particular object? Know that your guide can assist you with finding the answer you seek. When I count to three, you and your guide will float all the way back to the source event or the most significant event in your past that will give you the answer to why you're so drawn to that object. Ready? One, floating back, back, back; two, further and further, you're almost there; and three. Be there now. Float down into that early time and notice what you notice.

Where are you? Allow the first thought to pop into your mind. What year is this? As you take a look around or have an inner knowing, do you sense the object is near you? If so, where? In what capacity do you use this item? Can you become clear about this connection now? If not, go ahead and fast-forward to the moment that would best explain why you enjoy this object. Be there now. Very good.

What's happening? Why has your soul been drawn to this particular article? What lessons are you learning from it or what role does this play in your soul journey? Very good.

Now imagine you can float forward in time through other important events. Allow any other insights to emerge.

[PAUSE]

Very good. When you're ready, imagine you can float up, up, up, out of that event. From that perspective, imagine you can come to a higher understanding of these events. What lessons did you learn during this early time? How is this life-time affecting your current incarnation? How did you utilize that object in those early times and how are you using that object now? Or are you? Perhaps the object simply serves to remind you of something from the deep past. If so, what? And why is it so important for your soul to recall that during your present lifetime? Allow all these answers to easily flow to you now. If needed, know your guide can explain any further helpful details you may need.

[PAUSE]

When you're ready, take your guide's hand and imagine the two of you can float all the way down, down, down, back through the clouds, and go back into the room where you started.

Thank your guide for helping today and notice as they float away. Turn and go back out the door, back to where you started. Be there now. Still surrounded by the healing golden light, allow that light to remain with you now and always. When I count back from five, you will return, feeling awake, refreshed, and better than you felt before. Ready? Five, grounded, centered, and balanced; four, processing all of this information in your dreams tonight, so by tomorrow morning, you will be fully integrated into this new energy; three, recalling the lessons you received today so you can use them in your current experience; two, driving safely and being safe always; and one, you're back!

Were you able to connect with an object? Did the results surprise you? Did you uncover details about anything you're using now, or did you simply need to recall an earlier time for some higher purpose and learning? Awesome work!

Past Life Regression to the Source Event with an Artifact

By now, it should be quite apparent that artifacts in museums have energies that can undoubtedly cause you to have strong blasts from the past. In this exercise, you're going to go back to a source event to see why you were so affected by something you saw on exhibit.

EXERCISE

Settle into your comfortable chair or space and relax. Close your eyes and take a deep breath in through your nose. Breathe in healing, peace, and relaxation, and exhale any tensions. Allow a loving light to move through your body from head to toe. Notice now that this light is helping you relax even more than before as it forms a ball of healing golden light around you. Very good.

There's a doorway in front of you. You may see the door, feel it, or simply allow yourself to acknowledge that door, the same door you've been through before. When I count to three, that door will open, and you will float inside your special healing place. Ready? One, two, and three. Open the door and go inside that room now. Feel the loving vibrations and the supportive energy as you deepen this feeling of peace within every single cell in your being. Very good.

Now notice your angel or spirit guide is approaching you. Allow yourself to really feel the tremendous love they have for you. They've been with you since the beginning of eternity, so they're a trusted, supportive friend who is here today to assist you with this very important work. Hold their hand, and the two of you will begin to float. You're lifting higher and higher and higher, up, up, up, floating out of the ceiling of your special space and going higher and higher into the clouds until you find yourself once again floating over today.

Ask your special guide a question: Why did I have such a reaction to the particular artifact I encountered? Allow an artifact you experienced in the past to float into your memory, into your mind's eye, then take the angel by the hand again as the two of you begin to float. Floating back, back, back, you will go past your current lifetime into the very early past. Allow your guide to help you go all the way back in time to the actual source event to explain your fascination with this item. On the count of three, you will arrive at the source event. Ready? One, two, three. Be there now.

Floating over this early time, imagine you and your guide are floating down, down, down into those events. Be there now. Notice what's happening. What year is this? Note the first thought that pops into your mind? Where are you? Are you alone or with others? Do you sense the artifact from your current lifetime is in use during these early times? If so, what is it used for and how are you involved? Take your time to gather all you need from this experience, and if necessary, allow your soul to fast-forward through various events during these early times so you can fully understand what's happening.

[PAUSE]

Very good. Now take that information and energy with you as you and your guide lift up, up, up, over those early times. Your guide can help you gain greater understanding of these events. Why were you so attracted to that artifact? What benefit is this recognition bringing to your current experience in the present day? How can you use this information to enhance your life journey or to assist others?

[PAUSE]

When you're ready, you and your guide will hold hands and float all the way back, down through the clouds, carrying all this new wisdom and insight with you as you arrive back in your sacred space where you began. Thank your loving guide for their assistance and watch while they float away. Turn now and go back out where you began, closing that door behind you. In a moment, you will come back feeling lighter, more energized, and filled with new wisdom. Ready? Five, grounded, centered, and balanced; four, knowing that you may receive more insights in your dreams tonight, so by tomorrow morning, you will be fully integrated into this new learning; three, being safe always; two, grounded and centered; and one, you're back!

I wish we could sit down together so I could hear what happened on that journey. There's no doubt when you're attracted to various museum artifacts that the magnetism is happening for a reason. I hope you gained more insight into the depth of your soul. Awesome!

Past Life Regression to the Source Event with an Antique

I would assume that every person alive has been around antiques at some point during their life experience. Whether you visited one of those antique malls stuffed with old items or went to a flea market or simply visited the home of a dear grandparent, you may have been affected by something you encountered there.

If possible, think of one of those times or pull out your notes from the previous section before beginning this journey. Another option would be to simply take the regression and see what emerges in your mind's eye that perhaps you've forgotten about over the years. Either way, I know you will find this an interesting and informative process as it reveals a lot about your soul and your journey through your many lifetimes.

Another interesting thing to consider is the fact that antiques only need to be over twenty-five years old. Shocking, right? Imagine my surprise to find many of the things I grew up with have been antiques for quite some time. While it may seem like yesterday, time does indeed fly! For that reason, you may want to remain super open to what emerges for you in this process.

Settle in, and let's get ready!

EXERCISE

Finding yourself back in your comfortable and nurturing space, close your eyes and start to breathe. As you've done before, allow the healing light to flow through the top of your head, into your neck and shoulders, moving through your arms, hands, and down through your spine, into your heart and stomach, your lungs, and into your legs and feet. Know that this healing light is removing any tensions and concerns you may have and allowing those to flow out of the body. Very good.

The loving light is surrounding you by three feet or more in all directions. You find yourself floating in this protective shield of light, and you know that here, only that which is of your highest good can come through. See, feel, or imagine your familiar doorway. Go ahead and step through that door and be inside your sacred space. Your guide is here to greet you.

Thank your guide for helping you yet again and take their hand as the two of you float out of that sacred space and find yourselves in the clouds. You're floating up, and the higher up you float, the more relaxed you feel. The energy feels so wonderful and relaxed. You notice how easy it is to float away, and you go to a space so high in the sky, you are now hovering over the present day. As you float there, imagine an antique you've encountered in your current life can either float out in front of you or emerge in your mind's eye. Notice the first item that pops into your mind. Very good.

Gaze back in the direction of your past. Your guide is about to assist you in traveling back to the true source event that will show you why you're so attracted to the antique that has emerged at this time. Ready? Floating back in time, further and further, go all the way back to the earliest time or the source event that will give you the most insights into this antique. On the count of three, you will arrive. One, two, and three, you're there! Be there now.

Float down into this early time. What year is this? Where are you? Fast-forward easily through various events until you encounter the reason why this particular antique has emerged. Notice that now. Take your time and continue to flow through the events that will fully explain your connection with this antique.

[PAUSE]

Good work! Now float up, up, up, out of this event. Allow your guide to help you notice an energetic cord connecting you with this antique. When I count to three, your guide is going to cut the cord between you and the item using a beautiful pair of golden scissors. Ready? One, two, three—cutting that cord now. Healing light is flooding over you, transforming this energy and lifting you and your angel higher and higher and higher. Floating in the clouds, allow your angel to discover the answers to important questions. Why were you drawn to this antique at this point on your life journey? What lessons did you learn from this? How can you utilize this information to enhance your present incarnation? Allow this information to easily flow in so you have full understanding.

[PAUSE]

Very nice. Hold your guide's hand as the two of you return to the sacred space where you started. Bringing all that loving light down, down, down, back through the clouds, you land inside that lovely room. Thank your guide for assisting you today as they float or walk away. Turn and go back through the door. In a moment, you will return feeling lighter, brighter, and better than before. Five, grounded, centered, and balanced; four, driving and being safe always in everything you do; three, noticing information that emerges in your dreams so you can take note of these important details upon awakening tomorrow; two; one, and you're back!

You did it again! Wonderful job! The journey is all the more meaningful when you can uncover the reasons why the information is emerging. There's always a good reason why different scenarios come up when they do, and, typically, they're there to help with the particular place you find yourself in at any moment in life.

Past Life Regression to the Global Location of a Gem or Stone

No doubt gems and stones can bring us closer to various places on Earth. You're drawn to stones because they bring you closer to the places you loved or to the locations you most need to heal from during your life journey, and gemstones help you so you don't need to go flying around the globe in order to bring about real change.

For this next regression journey, you may want to locate a special stone to work with. If you don't have the one that first comes to mind, just think of it in your mind's eye before starting. If nothing is emerging now, ask that your highest good be revealed, and see what floats in as you go on this regression to the place in the world that is the source of a long-forgotten memory from your very early past.

EXERCISE

If possible, hold the gemstone while you take this journey and go relax in the space you've created for healing and personal reflection. Close your eyes and allow yourself to fully unwind and relax.

Allow the healing light to flow through your body, and know that each time you breathe in through your nose, you are deepening your sense of peace and rest, allowing important thoughts to emerge that will be for your highest good. While you breathe, you realize that the loving light you have come to know and understand has fully surrounded you in a healing embrace. You are safe and fully able to explore the depths of your soul.

Open your door and cross into the special space where you know you are fully supported. Meet your guide and go together into the clouds, leaving the world behind. Know that the higher you and your guide float, the more open and relaxed and ready to receive divine support and insights you will become. You and your guide have now floated so high, you are gently existing above today. Allow a gem or stone to emerge in your mind's eye or watch while it floats in front of you. Ask your guide, "Where does this stone come from, and how am I connected to this area of the world?"

Your guide will now take you there. The two of you float over your past, beyond your current lifetime, to the real source of your connection with this stone and the place where it comes from on Earth. On the count of three, you and your guide will arrive. Ready? One, two, and three—you will be there now!

Where are you in the world? What year is this? Move through the important events of this early time and understand why you're so drawn to that energy. Notice any souls there whom you may also have current life connections with and allow yourself to experience the most important events during this early time.

[PAUSE]

Very good. Now float up and out of these experiences and find yourself floating over this early time. What lessons did you learn there? Why has your soul chosen to be so attracted to that location in your current lifetime? How is this place on the planet contributing to your soul growth? Allow your guide to tell you anything else that is helpful for you to know at this time.

[PAUSE]

When you're ready, take your guide's hand and float down quickly as you find yourself easily returning to your special place. Thank your guide for once again gifting you with such valuable insights into your soul. Watch while they float or fly away and go back out the door where you started. Be there now, still surrounded by loving light. When I count down from five, you'll come back, feeling better than ever before. Five, grounded, centered, and balanced; four, continuing to process this information in your dreams tonight, so by tomorrow morning, you will be fully integrated into your new way of being, deeply appreciating various parts of our amazing planet; three, always finding yourself safe in every activity; two, grounded to the earth; and one, you're back!

Where did you go? Had you ever considered such a deep connection to the place that emerged during this journey? Allow more insights to float in over the next several days, and take notes if needed. Awesome!

Past Life Healing from Geographical Supretrovie

This exercise will help you access the truth behind any challenging geographical places you visited that either felt familiar or where you were adversely affected. During such trips, you may have experienced incredibly strange sensations, or perhaps a little movie played in your mind. The modern surroundings may have faded into something you'd never seen before or hadn't seen in hundreds or even thousands of years. In other words, the past life memory emerged, but without context. You now will go to gain healing and understanding of the memory you've already experienced. As you saw with the case histories, one of the main reasons to do a regression is to uncover unpleasant situations and heal them so you can return to certain locales if you so choose and experience greater levels of peace and happiness doing so. Ready to find out the deeper details about places your soul found familiar? Let's get started!

EXERCISE

Sit down in a comfortable chair with your feet on the floor and your hands on your lap. Take a deep, relaxing breath as you close your eyes, and imagine a beam of pure white light going down through the top of your head.

Allow the white light to move in through the top of your head, going down, down, down, into your eyes, your nose, into your jaw, and down, down, down into your neck. Allow the white light to heal you, and relax you, as it moves down, down, down, into your shoulders, into your elbows, your wrists, your hands, and down, down, down into your fingertips. The loving light continues to move down into your shoulders, through your shoulder blades. Feel your shoulders relax as that white light continues to move down, down, down, through your back, into your heart, moving into your stomach. Very good!

Feel the light moving into your lungs. Go ahead now and take a deep breath in through your nose, breathing in love and light, and exhaling tension and concern. Very good. With each breath you take, you're feeling more and more relaxed as that white light moves down, down, down, into your legs, moving into your thighs, your knees, your calves, into your ankles and down, down, down into the soles of your feet.

Imagine this beautiful white light is pouring through, removing any concerns as you allow tension to leave the body and travel down, down, down, through your legs, and down, down, down, out the soles of your feet and into the earth. As those tensions move into the earth, see them transforming into a healing light that goes into the earth, healing and blessing the planet. Very good.

The light is becoming stronger and stronger, so powerful. It begins to pour out of your heart, creating a beautiful golden ball of light that surrounds you by about three feet in all directions. Feel yourself floating inside the healing warmth of this golden light as it surrounds you and heals you. Just know that within this golden ball of light, only your highest good can come through.

Now imagine a doorway in front of you. See it, feel it, or just allow yourself to have an inner knowing that the doorway is there. Very good.

Walk or float through that door now. You find yourself inside a beautiful room. Look around the room and notice what's there. See the beautiful surroundings and feel the peaceful energy and the good vibrations of this special place as you begin to explore. See what you see, hear what you hear. Very good.

Enjoying the peaceful energy of this space, feeling safe, relaxed, and at ease, imagine a beautiful being of pure love and light floating down in front of you. You can see this guide, feel their loving energy, or just have an inner knowing that the guide is with you now. Very good. Imagine this guide knows everything about you, your soul, and your soul's journey. Feel the unconditional love and high regard your guide has for you. As you experience the amazing energy of this guide, you come to an understanding that this being has been with you forever. They know every single thing there is to know about you, and today, they've come to assist you in accessing important information about your soul and your soul's journey.

Take your guide's hand as the two of you begin to float. Float through the ceiling of the beautiful room and find yourself floating up, up, up, higher and higher into the clouds; notice that the higher up you float, the more relaxed you'll be. Very good. You have now floated so high in the sky that as you gaze down, you notice a beautiful ray of sunshine below you. This ray of light represents time, and you and your loving guide are gently floating over today. Be there now, floating over the present day. Notice how peaceful and relaxed you feel. Go ahead now and glance out in the direction of your future. Notice how bright the sunshine is in your future. Then turn and face your past. As you do, the sunshine is getting lighter and lighter, brighter and brighter. So bright, so wonderful. Very good.

Take your guide by the hand and imagine the two of you can glance into the past. Begin to float now. Floating further and further into the past, notice that the further back you go, the earlier the time will be. Imagine you and your guide are floating back... over your soul's history... further and further... back... into the past, going way, way, way, way back, to a very early time that will be for your highest good:

a time that is connected to a memory you had in your current life of the places you lived before.

Go back to a time that will give you the most insight into the place that caused the memories to surface.

You will reach the appropriate place when I count to three. Ready? One, floating back into the past; two, further and further; and three. You're there! Be there now, and imagine your guide stops, and the two of you can float down, down, down, into that event. Be there now and notice what's happening.

Where are you? Notice the first thing that pops into your mind. What year is this? Are you a man or a woman? What are you wearing? Look at your feet. What kind of shoes are you wearing? How do you feel?

If you cannot bring these details to mind, imagine your guide can tell you what you are wearing or that you can have an inner knowing or gut feeling. Good job!

Are you alone or with other people? If you're with other people, who are they? Notice their relationship to you. Imagine you can fast-forward to the next most significant event in your life where you are with other people whom you know. Be there now. What's happening?

Who's with you? As you experience the energy of the other people there, is there anyone you know from your current life? Feel the energy and notice if anyone feels familiar. Maybe, maybe not. If yes, what lessons did the two of you learn that you are still experiencing in your current life? Very good.

Now imagine you can float to the very last day of that life. Be there now. Notice how you pass into spirit and do that now. Floating up, up, up, out of that body, out of that life. Your guide is with you now as you float higher and higher and higher. Float into that beautiful, peaceful space between lives where you're safe and secure.

Imagine your guide can help you answer some important questions. What lessons did you learn in that life? Why did your soul choose to return to that place in your current life? What are you learning or accessing by doing so? How does that information relate to your current life? Very good!

Now, from that space high in the clouds, take your guide by the hand and float all the way back to the present day, allowing all events between then and now to heal and transform in light of this new information. Be there now, floating over today. Hold your guide's hand and float down, down, down, back through the clouds, through the ceiling of the beautiful room where we started. Be there now. Very good!

Thank your guide for being here today and watch as they float back through the ceiling.

Say goodbye and know you can return here at any time to meet your guide and receive assistance. Go ahead now and walk back through the door where you began. Close the door behind you and find yourself standing right back where we started. Good job! You're still surrounded by that golden ball of light, safe and protected, totally secure, knowing that within this golden light, only that which is of your highest good can come through. When I count from five, you will come back, feeling awake, refreshed, and better than you did before.

Five, grounded, centered, and balanced; four, continuing to process this information in your dreams tonight, so by tomorrow morning, you will be fully integrated into this new energy and information; three, driving safely and being safe in all activities; two, grounded, centered, and balanced; and one, you're back!

Welcome back! How do you feel? You may want to make notes in your journal, and you'll want to keep that nearby in case more insights occur to you in your dreams. Great job!

Past Life Healing from Artifact- or Antique-Induced Supretrovie

We talked about artifacts and antiques and the information about your soul they can unearth during a previous regression exercise. But what happens if those insights come to you out of the blue while you're touring a museum, for example? This next process will help you finish up and find answers for what happened and why the experience affected you. Let's get started!

EXERCISE

Sit in your special space. Close your eyes and breathe. Allow the healing light to surround you as you walk through the door and go into the beautiful room.

Your guide is there waiting. Notice your guide has a television or a big screen set up and invites you to relax as you enjoy a special movie. Imagine your guide is about to show you a movie that will better explain the reaction you experienced from either an antique or artifact you encountered in your waking life. Know that this film will explore the details about your prior connections to this item or items and will explain all you need to know for your higher learning. Ready? The guide is starting that film now. Imagine you can either watch the screen or hear a narrator telling you all about this connection. Notice what you notice and take your time.

[PAUSE]

The film is stopping, and your guide is turning to you to help you with important questions you've come here to ask: In what way were you connected to this artifact or antique?

Why did you have such a reaction to it during your current incarnation? What lessons are you learning from encountering that item again in the present experience? How will you best use this information to create greater peace and happiness in your life? Take your time and get solid answers to these questions, and feel free to ask your guide anything else you'd like to know.

[PAUSE]

Wonderful! Now thank your guide for once again being so very helpful. Stand and go through the door where you came in, back to where you started. In a moment, when I count down from five, you will come back feeling better than ever. Five, grounded, centered, and balanced; four, continuing to process this information in your dreams tonight, so by tomorrow morning, you are fully integrated into this new self-understanding and awareness; three, being safe always; two, continuing to remain grounded to the earth; and one, you're coming back!

Were you able to find the answers you needed? Amazing! Feel free as usual to do this exercise again on other items you've encountered through the years. Each time, you will likely get a new result. Also keep track of important soul patterns or information that may yield clues into some of your deeper life lessons and soul gifts.

Past Life Healing from a Gemstone- or Mineral-Induced Supretrovie

Earlier in the book, you read about people who had strong blasts from their past lives after being in the presence of particular gems and stones. This may have even happened to you, and if you're like me, you might not have noticed before. In this exercise, you'll have a chance to uncover the deeper meaning behind your connection to the gem and mineral kingdom and learn more about yourself in the process.

If possible, you may want to hold the gem you're curious about, or if this incident happened while you were out somewhere, you can recall the gem you'd like to learn more about or allow one to bubble up in your mind as we go along. Either way, you're bound to uncover some interesting information about yourself. Ready? Let's begin.

EXERCISE

Comfortable and relaxed in your favorite place, hold the stone you are curious about in your hands and close your eyes. If you don't have the stone with you, that's okay. Go ahead and close your eyes and breathe. Absorbing peace, healing, and love, allow yourself to become more and more relaxed with each breath you take. Very nice. Notice how easy it is to surround yourself with a golden, protective, healing light. Very good.

Now walk or float through the doorway into your comfortable room. As you enter the room, your guide is there to greet you, and you can find a comfortable space where you can sit and have a conversation about the past. Imagine that with the help of your guide, you can easily recall a memory from your past when a gem made a stronger-than-normal impression on you. Perhaps you loved the stone, or perhaps you had a deep dislike emerge. Allow the first thought to float into your mind. If you need help recalling this early time, imagine your guide can tell you about these memories or you can have an inner knowing.

Once your memory emerges, talk to your guide and ask an important question: "Was this feeling connected to a past life? Yes or no?" Allow the first thought you have to float into your mind.

Now notice your guide has brought you a video screen. In just a moment, your guide will play a movie on this screen that will give you more detailed insights into your connection with the stone you're thinking about today. Ready? Your guide turns on the video. Go ahead now and watch this film. What's happening? Who is in this movie? How do you feel watching it? As you connect with one of the characters in the film, imagine you can notice that this is you in a past life. Who were you? Were you a man or woman? What happened in the film that gave you such a strong reaction, and how is that affecting you now? Take your time as the film plays and notice all you can or need to experience at this time.

[PAUSE]

Very nice. Now ask your guide to help you understand the lessons you learned in this early time. Why did you encounter this stone again in your current incarnation, and why is that important to you now? Allow your guide to show you the final part of the film. Take your time to gain all the information and detail you need.

[PAUSE]

Very good! Take a moment to thank your guide for assisting you today. When you're ready, stand up and walk back through the door, closing that door behind you. You're back, right where you started. Be there now. In a moment, you will come back feeling better than ever. Ready? Five, grounded, centered, and balanced; four, continuing to process this information in your dreams tonight, so by tomorrow morning, you will be integrated fully into this new energy of your stone or gem; three, driving and being careful and safe in every activity; two; one, and you're back!

Were you able to watch the video? Did anything surprising emerge? Write down any details, and you may find that you have a new energy around that particular stone the next time you encounter it. You may also want to do some research about the stone itself and what part of the world it comes from. Think about that location and see how you can learn more to enhance your healing. Awesome work!

Past Life Healing and Discovery from a Close Encounter Supretrovie

Have you ever gazed into someone's eyes and felt you'd been whisked away to times long gone? Did you have a loving feeling for a stranger or an instant trepidation toward someone you knew you could never trust? It's time to get to the bottom of such feelings.

You may or may not consciously recall if or when this happened. Whether you recall the encounter or not, in this next process, you will go into a deeper state of peace and relaxation so those dormant memories can emerge and you can finally have answers about the strongest connections you've felt during your life journey. Ready? Great!

EXERCISE

Go ahead and sit down in your relaxing space and close your eyes. Breathe in a peaceful, healing breath as a loving light moves through you from head to toe. Allow this light to relax your mind, your jaw and neck, your shoulders. Breathe that light into your lungs as it travels through your heart and stomach to the base of your spine. Know that with every breath, you are becoming more and more peaceful and relaxed. The light is moving quickly from head to feet, pouring out the soles of your feet. Imagine you can let any tensions and concerns float through your feet and let those go down into the earth. As that energy moves into the planet, imagine it is immediately transformed into a wonderful healing light that sends love to all people, places, and things on Earth. Very nice.

Feel that love extend now to you. The light moves around you, surrounding you with a golden glow of love and peace.

Imagine you can easily float in this golden bubble of love, and know that within this space, you are safe and protected always.

Now recognize how easy it is to see your doorway. Walk or float through that same door to the safe and sacred space where you've been so many times before. Be there now, inside your special room. Very good. Your guide is waiting for you. They're saying hello to you. Feel the unconditional love they have for you. Go ahead and take their hand as the two of you begin to float. Up, up, up, out of the ceiling of your special sacred space, you and your guide are moving higher and higher and higher, up, up, up into the clouds. Notice that the higher up you float, the more relaxed you feel. Nice job!

You and your guide are now floating over today. Be there now. Float over today. Allow the memory of a person from your current life to bubble up in your mind. Imagine it's easy to think about a person you met whom you had an instant connection to, a person whom you felt you'd known before. Notice the first person who bubbles up into your mind. This could be someone you're incredibly fond of, or it may be someone you distrust. Either way, know that you are still so safe and secure and that your guide is with you always and that all is well. On the count of three, imagine you can have the person emerge in your mind. Ready? One, two, and three! They're there! Allow your guide to tell you who they are right now. Very good.

Next, hold that image in your mind's eye as you and your guide gaze in the direction of your past. In a moment, you and your guide will float back to the true source event and the original moment or the most significant time when you knew this person who felt so familiar to you. Ready? One, floating back in time; two, further and further beyond your current lifetime; and three, you're there! Be there now!

Surrounded by light with your guide by your side, float down into this early event. Be there now. Notice what's happening. Where are you? What year is this? Notice the first thoughts that pop into your mind. What's happening?

[PAUSE]

Imagine you can move through these events until you find yourself with the person you thought about earlier and discover that connection. Who were they to you? What lessons did the two of you come to learn about over these lifetimes? Why did you meet again in your current life? Take your time to notice all you can.

[PAUSE]

Very good. Now imagine you can float up, up, up out of that life, and float over that early time. Notice there's an energetic cord of light coming out of your stomach area and connecting you with this person from the past. Even if this connection felt good, in a moment, your guide will help you cut those cords to create either a stronger, cleaner bond with that energy or to release it altogether so you will no longer be affected by that energy. Ready? Three, two, one—cutting that cord now. Your guide has cut the cord with the golden scissors, and a white, healing light is pouring forth, healing and cleansing you and all souls involved in these events from this very early time. Imagine all parties involved are becoming lighter and lighter and lighter and brighter and brighter than ever before. Very nice. Allow that light to lift you up, higher and higher so you're floating over those events, and while holding your guide's hand, imagine the two of you will float back toward today and the present moment, but only as quickly as all events between this very early time can heal and become even lighter than before.

When I count back from three, you will be floating over today once more. Three, so relaxed; two, allowing this healing light to transform all people involved in this early time; and one, you're floating over today. Gaze back into the past and notice now how much lighter and brighter the past is thanks to this amazing healing.

Take your guide by the hand as the two of you float down, down, down and back through the clouds. Come all the way back and float through the ceiling of the beautiful room where you started. Thank your loving guide for assisting you today. Imagine they float or fly away as you turn to go back through the door you initially walked through. Walk through that door now. Close the door. Find yourself back where you started.

When I count back from five, you will return. Ready? Five, grounded, centered, and balanced; four, continuing to receive the positive effects from this light and healing through the rest of your life; three, knowing you will be fully integrated into this healing by tomorrow morning; two, being safe always; and one, you're back!

Nice job! Were you finally able to come to terms with the connection you had with this other person? Did the situation need to be healed, or did you have a positive connection? The cord cutting process is one that can (and I would say *should*) be done even in the most positive situations, because it is like sending a huge cosmic blessing to the other person and saying that no matter what went on in the past, you want things to be even better than before. One interesting by-product of any cord cutting is the fact that the person will often want to reconnect with you once you do that, so pay attention these next coming days, weeks, and even months. Your personal blast from the past may come calling sooner than you think!

And as per usual, remember to take note of important thoughts or feelings you had that might help you down the road. Wonderful work!

Summing Up

I hope the past life journeys have given you food for thought and helpful clues about your journey through life. Remember to pull this book out periodically during different times and chapters of your life to receive new insights relevant to the place you're at on your life path, because each time you do these processes, you're liable to get different results that are meaningful to a particular moment in time. Namaste!

CONCLUSION

Thank you for going on this journey with me. This book has given me the opportunity to further consider the many amazing souls I've met over the years and explore my philosophies on why past life regression is so important for reasons other than recalling who we were in prior lives. I'm more convinced than ever that residue from our past bombards us every moment of our lives, whether we realize it or not. Our soul craves familiarity, and we prearrange divine appointments with certain people in very specific places and times to finish up old business and complete aspects of our soul learning plan.

Travel is never coincidental. The soul calls us to faraway places for reasons we cannot possibly understand. If we listen carefully, the most amazing stories begin to unfold as we ultimately come to know ourselves better. When travel isn't possible, artifacts, objects, gems, stones, and even what may seem like a chance encounter can also serve to enhance our soul journey and offer a transformational state of remembrance on the path toward healing.

I hope this exploration will help you consciously choose to become more aware of why you're participating in various activities or traveling to the locations you're drawn to visit.

Such encounters might seem either totally random or like conscious choices. Perhaps instead our Higher Selves, our spirit guides, and our soul helpers are leading us down familiar roads to enable us to complete the contracts we've made in the past. Each detail of our life journey might be playing a far bigger part in our daily lives than we ever deemed possible.

By fearlessly exploring the phenomenon of Supretrovie and choosing to work through challenging times to gain a wider and more enlightened perspective on reality, we not only enrich our own lives, but we also help the other souls whom we agreed to go on this journey through space and time with to complete their own life lessons. Likewise, once such challenges are healed through conscious awareness, we can return to places that were once the source of suffering and begin anew with a refreshed perspective of people, situations, and places. That level of awareness shifts our past karma into loving dharma as we move forward with a more tolerant perspective of everything and everyone around us.

I hope this writing gave you pause to think about your own soul journeys and experiences. Remember that even a trip to a local market can become instantly magical if you're open to recognizing the divine connection unfolding through each step of our lives. Remain ever-open by allowing your soul knowing to work miracles in your life. You'll be amazed by what will happen, whom you'll meet, and what you'll discover as incredible adventures open to you. Know I'm wishing you well on your life path now and always. Namaste!

BIBLIOGRAPHY

De Lisser, Herbert G. *The White Witch of Rose Hall.* New York: Macmillan Education, 1929, 1982.

Dictionary.com. "Anamnesis." Accessed May 22, 2020. https://www.dictionary.com/browse/anamnesis?s=t.

Encyclopaedia Britannica. "Anamnesis." Last modified June 16, 2016. https://www.britannica.com/art/anamnesis.

Encyclopaedia Britannica. "Kilauea." Accessed May 22, 2020. https://www.britannica.com/place/Kilauea.

History.com Editors. "Ming Dynasty." Last modified January 10, 2018. https://www.history.com/topics/ancient-china/ming-dynasty.

Jowett, Benjamin. *MENO by Plato 380 BC.* New York: C. Scribner's Sons, 1871.

———. *PHAEDO by Plato 360 BC.* New York: C. Scribner's Sons, 1871.

———. *PHAEDRUS by Plato 360 BC*. New York: C. Scribner's Sons, 1871.

Jung, C. G. *Collected Papers on Analytical Psychology*. London: Balliere, Tindall and Cox, 1920.

Lenz, Frederick. *Lifetimes—True Accounts of Reincarnation*. New York: The Bobbs-Merrill Company, 1979.

Plato, John M. Cooper, and G. M. A. Grube. *Five Dialogues: Euthyphro, Apology, Crito, Meno, Phaedo*. Indianapolis, IN: Hackett Publishing Company, 2002.

World Heritage List. "Gorham's Cave Complex." *Unesco*, 2016. https://whc.unesco.org/en/list/1500/.

Wotton, Chris. "Death Railway: History of the Bridge on the River Kwai." *The Culture Trip*, July 17, 2018. https://theculturetrip.com /asia/thailand/articles/bridge-on-the-river-kwai-a-place-to -remember-thailands-past/.

To Write to the Author

If you wish to contact the author or would like more information about this book, please write to the author in care of Llewellyn Worldwide Ltd. and we will forward your request. Both the author and the publisher appreciate hearing from you and learning of your enjoyment of this book and how it has helped you. Llewellyn Worldwide Ltd. cannot guarantee that every letter written to the author can be answered, but all will be forwarded. Please write to:

Shelley A. Kaehr, PhD
℅ Llewellyn Worldwide
2143 Wooddale Drive
Woodbury, MN 55125-2989

Please enclose a self-addressed stamped envelope for reply, or $1.00 to cover costs. If outside the U.S.A., enclose an international postal reply coupon.

Many of Llewellyn's authors have websites with additional information and resources. For more information, please visit our website at http://www.llewellyn.com.